AF504548

F' YOU FIBRO

How I Found Happy

by

M. E. Nesser

DORRANCE
PUBLISHING CO
EST. 1920
PITTSBURGH, PENNSYLVANIA 15238

The contents of this work, including, but not limited to, the accuracy of events, people, and places depicted; opinions expressed; permission to use previously published materials included; and any advice given or actions advocated are solely the responsibility of the author, who assumes all liability for said work and indemnifies the publisher against any claims stemming from publication of the work.

All Rights Reserved
Copyright © 2024 by M.E. Nesser

No part of this book may be reproduced or transmitted, downloaded, distributed, reverse engineered, or stored in or introduced into any information storage and retrieval system, in any form or by any means, including photocopying and recording, whether electronic or mechanical, now known or hereinafter invented without permission in writing from the publisher.

Dorrance Publishing Co
585 Alpha Drive
Pittsburgh, PA 15238
Visit our website at *www.dorrancebookstore.com*

ISBN: 979-8-89211-072-3
eISBN: 979-8-89211-570-4

Definition of Fibromyalgia

Fibromyalgia is a disorder characterized by widespread musculoskeletal pain accompanied by fatigue, sleep, memory and mood issues. Researchers believe that fibromyalgia amplifies painful sensations by affecting the way your brain processes pain signals.

Mayo Clinic

M.E.'s Definition of Fibromyalgia

An obscure pain in my ass.

M.E. Nesser

TABLE OF CONTENTS

FOREWORD

I am one of those Type A personalities that would drive most of you bonkers. I'm not happy unless I'm being productive—or should I say ridiculously over productive? There are so many sides to my personality that you'd marvel at all the shit I have going on in my life. I am the proud mother of three, grandmother to one, and the blessed wife to a man for over thirty-six years. I own three beauty salons, do an exorbitant amount of social media advertising for all of my passions and businesses, write fiction and nonfiction books (such as this motivational memoir), write random articles in various publications, own real estate in New York and Florida, hold mortgages for individuals, cook like a gourmet chef, exercise daily, do all the accounting for our lives and still find time to travel, have lots of sex, and, lastly, enjoy my life. I get more done before nine in the morning than most people get done in an entire day. And the kicker is that I've been suffering from fibromyalgia since I was thirteen years old. So, you have to be wondering, if this chick has this bizarre disease, how the hell does she do it all? That's what this book is all about. I am here to change your life!

I have had difficulty sleeping for as long as I can remember. Yes, I could bitch about that and lie around feeling sorry for myself, but that isn't who I am. I could never lie around and feel sorry for myself, because that is such a blatant waste of time. I know that restorative sleep is important, but I just suck at it. Five hours straight and I feel like I can run a marathon. In fact, five hours is what I strive for every night. And that is five hours in a row, which rarely happens. Over the years I've convinced myself that sleep is overrated. I'm sure you've heard the old adage before that says, "I can sleep when I'm dead, right?" That's just one of my mantras.

Lying around watching a movie and simply hanging out are the kinds of activities that give this particular woman a lot of anxiety—and believe me, I've suffered from some major anxiety in the past. There are times when I think there is seriously something wrong with me because I have so many things that I want to do before I die that I've lost the ability to just hang out. I do make a concerted effort to decompress once in a while because I know that it is good for me. I indulge in baths, get regular massages, puzzles, practice meditation, and spend countless hours working on my food blog and writing. My husband and I also travel a lot more now that we are older because that has brought us a lot of joy. The crazy thing is that being busy makes me happy—even deliriously happy sometimes—and it also distracts me from the things in my life that aren't so great: specifically, my shitty body.

I'm not referring to the physical person you'd see if you met me; I'm talking about the inside of me, my bones, joints, tendons, and pretty much everything else that's under my skin. I believe the outside of me is pleasant looking, so if you looked at me, you'd think there was nothing wrong, and that is what I strive for. But that's where this whole fibro thing gets tricky.

It is truly the mechanical insides of my body that suck. Even though I'm your stereotypical Type A woman who thrives on busy work and has led a productive and successful life so far, I'm also a woman who has suffered from chronic pain her entire life. Yes, that is a fact and not an exaggeration. Living with constant pain for as long as I can remember has been a defining component of the woman I've become. Every day brings on a different challenge and overcoming adversity has made me very strong. Succumbing to my limitations has never been an option. I make a conscientious effort every day to work through my challenges and not let them consume me. What I learned early on is that keeping busy helps me ignore the pain or at least deal with it better. I am not the first one to admit that the pain really sucks, but being productive is rewarding, makes me feel better, and helps me tolerate the pain a little better.

I would be remiss if I didn't acknowledge my completely supportive and understanding husband Mark. Fortunately, I married a guy who is compassionate enough to love me through my shitty moods and continuous and relentless maladies. He also knows better than to coddle me, because, frankly, that would piss me off. He will rub my neck or help me when I have muscle weakness or am not strong enough to complete a task, but he never criticizes me or makes me feel weak, and for that, I will always be eternally grateful. His strength has given me the ammunition to stay strong and stay positive regardless of how I feel. I came to the realization a long time ago that succumbing to the negative shit in your life is an absolute waste of time, and fortunately I married someone who gets it.

I do my best to be positive about my condition because staying positive keeps me sane. I really wasn't kidding before; I have lived a lifetime filled with chronic pain, which means I feel pain all of the time. Sometimes it is mild, and there are other times it's like the worst fucking migraine of your life. My migraines aren't in my head, however. They're in my neck, knees, arms, hands… Believe me, this is not something that I am cavalier or flippant about and I have absolutely no reason or desire to exaggerate about how difficult living in my physical body has been. But I do know that I can offer you hope and guidance to help you deal with your pain, and that is the purpose of this book. I want to help you to be able to say "fuck you" to your pain, too.

For as long as I can remember, there has always been something in my body that has hurt. I have tried my hardest for the past forty-plus years to try and overcome this bizarre affliction that has plagued my insides. There has been a lot of trial and error involved as well numerous frustrating setbacks, but my fortitude has given me the ammunition to figure out the best way to deal with all the crap I've experienced. I know many of you can relate to my predicament because you have experienced a similar fate. On the other hand, I'm sure there are some of you who can't imagine that statement is completely true. How could a productive and outwardly happy member of society be in pain every day? I get your skepticism, especially since I look totally normal, and there are no visible signs of any ailment on my personage. That alone has to be one of the most frustrating aspects of being diagnosed with fibromyalgia;

in most cases, we look fine. Sometimes I think it would be so much easier for most people to empathize with my plight if I was missing a limb or looked like there was something gravely wrong with me. But I'm glad my pain isn't visible to others. I don't want pity; it's unproductive and focuses on the negative. My goal is to make every day happy—no matter what. Life is short, and I am here to live each day to the fullest. And if you think that sounds cliché, maybe you need a little more cliché in your life.

I try to live by a quote that means a lot to me and has for as long as I can remember from the song "Beautiful" by Carole King. She wrote, "You've got to wake up every morning with a smile on your face and show the world all the love in your heart." Now those are words to live by.

My primary goal for this book is to share my journey, make you smile, and offer you some hope. I'm confident that this is a way better goal than bitching about how shitty you or I feel. Bitching serves no purpose and isn't pretty on anyone, so let's try another approach.

At times, I may sound redundant when I talk about my pain or my quest to remain positive, but my hope is that if I reinforce my approach to this bizarre affliction, you will try to make your life better. Yes, there are times when I need to vent, because I am human like the rest of you, but I try to keep those moments to a minimum. I've learned that it's futile to blame anyone or anything for my predicament because—once again—it won't make me feel better. Moreover, I have discovered that whining about my issues only makes me feel worse, and what I strive for daily is to feel better. Besides, if I'm going to talk about wine, it will be of a red variety, particularly a Cabernet from California.

I guess this is the part where I should introduce myself. My name is Mary Elizabeth, but most people call me M.E. I'm a fifty-eight-year-old woman who has found writing to be very cathartic. At this point in my life, I'm relieved to have finally said bye-bye to menopause, which not only was a struggle in itself, it exasperated my challenges. The hot flashes, weight gain and mood swings were extremely annoying and it feels really good to have that stage of my life behind me so I could concentrate on finishing this memoir. There were several years during the height of menopause where it was too difficult to focus on this manuscript, so I was forced to put it on hold.

I have felt compelled to share my story for a few years now in the hopes of helping others cope with their pain. I am not a doctor, and I don't pretend to be. I'm just an educated woman who has been studying nutrition, health, fitness, and healing for decades and I feel confident that I can help—even if just a little. Orange may be the new black but living in pain has been my normal for as long as I can remember, and I'm here to remind you that you are not alone.

The first five chapters will give you an idea of the circumstances that triggered this condition and the different events that exasperated my symptoms over the years and eventually led to my diagnosis. You will also find out how I've learned to deal with it.

So, here's my story.

CHAPTER 1

GOOD MORNING MARY

"Time to get up," the familiar voice would say.

"I don't feel good," was the mantra that was becoming customary when I woke up in the morning.

"Take a shower, get dressed, and have a little breakfast and we'll see how you feel."

Ugh. My parents always made me get my ass out of bed no matter how crappy I felt. It was so annoying. They'd never just let me stay in bed and wallow in my misery. I wanted to, but it wasn't allowed. I was expected to get up and get moving no matter how much I whined about the malady of the moment. And boy there were a lot of maladies. Ironically, by the time I showered, got dressed, and ate something, I would feel a little better. Moving around did help. I hated to admit it, but they were always right. Besides, once I was dressed and ready for the day, it seemed ridiculous to get back into bed. Between their morning cheerfulness and words of nagging encouragement (I know that's an oxymoron, but it's the most accurate description of their approach to my bitching), I don't think I can ever remember missing a day of school.

Now that I've taken the time to reflect on how this journey started, I'm grateful for their insistence that I persevere regardless of how lousy I felt. If they weren't like that, I probably would have flunked out of middle school and ended up a real mess. I am convinced that their positive, ambitious personalities gave me the tools that I desperately needed to help me be as productive and successful as I am today.

Now that I'm grown and can look back at that time with more perspective, I realize the morning ritual between my parents and I saved me in more ways than I can even articulate. They were always such positive people. They taught me to look at the bright side of every aspect of my life even when things felt bleak, regardless of how I felt physically or emotionally. After taking a shower, getting dressed, and having breakfast, I always felt better. I may not have felt great, but I did feel better. Their encouragement allowed me to overcome how crappy I felt and gave me the power to deal with my physical issues in the most proactive ways possible.

Even though there were a lot of stressors in my life back then, I didn't think my complaints were psychosomatic, and I still don't. They may have been triggered by emotional or psychological problems, but they were real issues that caused me legitimate, physical pain. I may have been a prepubescent teen, but I know that I didn't embellish how I felt or make up what my body was experiencing. When I woke up in the morning, I did feel a lot of pain. I wasn't lying or exaggerating. God's honest truth was that I didn't feel good. My symptoms were real, even if there wasn't a rational explanation for them sometimes. At the tender age of thirteen, I was having frequent stomach aches, headaches, and overall body aches that were inexplicable and annoying as heck. Although my parents were the tough-love kind of folks with regard to my whining, I know they believed me. I wasn't a liar. My complaints were real. They just believed in the power of positive thinking and using a strong mindset to overcome adversity. When I look back on that time in my life, I realize their support and encouragement made me strong and gave me the power to overcome the variety of hardships in my life. Not only did they *give* me life, but they also saved my life as well.

But I was still confused by the awful feelings that were plaguing me. Sometimes I really doubted myself. Was I a moody, hypochondriac teenager, or was there something legitimately wrong with me? Sadly, it took twenty-two years for me to discover that I had a condition that was causing all of my physical problems. More importantly, I realized once and for all that I wasn't crazy. Believe me, there were times when I thought I was going nutty. Twenty-two years was a long time to not have an answer to my ongoing health concerns. It's a miracle that I didn't go a little bonkers. OK, maybe I'm a little cuckoo, but at least I'm cuckoo with a sense of humor.

CHAPTER 2

PRIVATE SCHOOL

When I was in the fourth grade, my parents asked me if I'd be interested in attending a private school the following year. It was an elite institution that was supported by a hefty tuition. I never remember hearing about scholarships, so I was pretty certain that every student came from affluent families. There was no elementary education offered by this school. The middle school housed students from the fifth to seventh grade, and the high school admitted students from the eighth to twelfth grade. The school transitioned from an all-male school to a coed one shortly before I planned to attend. It was actually my older siblings who suggested to my folks I go to a better school, and my parents agreed that it could be a good fit for me.

At the time, I was going to our local public school. Not only was I bored with the easy curriculum, but I was also frustrated by a few things that happened. There was one incident in particular that still sticks in my mind that I know was a catalyst for my decision to switch schools. Back then, the desks had a tabletop attached to the seat with the left side cut out so the students could sit down from that side. Since I was left-handed, I had to turn my body towards the right to rest my forearm on the desk so I could write legibly. I remember a time in the fourth grade when I was turned in my chair taking a test. The teacher yanked me from the room and accused me of cheating. I admit I was facing the student to the right, but that was only because I needed to rest my arm on the desk specifically designed for right-handed students so I could write the answers on the test. I was so embarrassed that day. The teacher humiliated me with her unfounded accusations. I wasn't cheating. I didn't have to. The test was easy for me, as they always were. I was confused, embarrassed, and outraged that this woman was accusing me of trying to see the student's paper next to me. This incident happened around the time that the private school discussion came up. For me, it was the final straw. If I passed the entrance exam, I was going to change schools the following year.

The only thing that caused me any hesitation about switching schools was leaving my best friend Karen who lived a few houses away from us. When we weren't at school, we spent pretty much every waking moment together. She was my very best friend in the whole world and had been for as long as I could remember, and I knew that once I changed schools, our relationship would change—and it did. But for some reason, I was willing to make the sacrifice because I was convinced that the public school was not for me. I wanted more out of life.

I was also extremely close with her sister, Suzy, who was mentally challenged. The three of us spent a lot of time together, and the thought of not seeing them regularly made me really sad. We made a pact to remain close, but sadly the new school made it nearly impossible to see each other very often, and our relationship was never the same once I started private school. It's funny because even as I'm editing this part, the thought of Karen and Suzy makes me smile. They were a very important part of my childhood, and I am grateful for the time we had together.

Suzy had a large impact on my life in many ways and I reflect on my experiences with her with such fondness, because I truly believe my association with her made me a better person.

There is something very endearing about children who are mentally challenged. We played together just as any normal child would, and I don't remember ever fighting or feeling annoyed because she was different from the rest of us. On the contrary, I wish more people were like Suzy. Unlike some two-faced, backstabbing kids I had to deal with at school, she was always honest and kind. It was amazing. She didn't have a mean bone in her body or understand the concept of hate. Her influence on me was profound.

My parents whole-heartedly agreed with my older brother and sister that it was a good idea for me to change schools, so when they approached me with the option, I was excited. This school was no joke, though. You didn't just pay the tuition, and voila, you were a part of this elite institution. I had to take an entrance exam to see if I was even smart enough to be accepted to the school. The test was going to take several hours to complete, and I had never taken a test that long before. The entire process was quite intimidating, but for some reason, I felt up to the challenge, because I desperately wanted a change. When that woman accused me of cheating, I knew I had to get the hell out of my current school. And to be honest, I was too humiliated to ever want to go back. Her accusation was tough on me, especially since it was unfounded.

If I did pass the entrance exam, my parents were adamant that it was *my* decision one way or another as to whether I attended this school or not. I think it was very open-minded of them to let me be part of the decision-making process, especially since I was only in the fourth grade at the time. As I said, I always found school to be boring and ridiculously easy and when I was presented with the opportunity to go to a private school, I realized that I was ready for something new. Even though I was very young, I was looking forward to having a challenge academically. I remember telling my folks that I'd rather be a C student at a private school than an A student at that public school, because, for some reason, I knew that the private school would give me more opportunities in life. That was when they arranged for me to take the entrance exam.

When I walked into the gymnasium, I remember feeling sick to my stomach. There were so many kids waiting to take the test that I felt overwhelmed and claustrophobic. It's ironic that I still suffer from claustrophobia to this very day, but that's a whole other story that we will save for later. To begin with, I didn't know anybody, and that was terrifying. Even though I really wanted to go to the school, I immediately felt out of place. The school had an incredibly prestigious reputation, which was a new experience for me, but I knew this was the kind of school that could better prepare me for college one day. Besides, I always knew I wanted to be successful, and I was confident that this place could help me do just that.

It's hard for me to put into words how strongly I felt like an outsider that morning. To this day, I'm not sure if something happened while I waited to enter the gymnasium that made me feel so uncomfortable, but I clearly remember the uneasy feeling in my gut. While we waited in the library that was located outside of the gym, I remember there was a video playing on a projector in the area that was talking about reproduction, which seemed odd, inappropriate, and fairly disconcerting. It showed the tadpole connecting with the eggs… Regardless, more than anything, I remember how scared and out of place I felt.

Most of the other kids waiting to take the test knew one another, were dressed differently, and didn't acknowledge me at all. It was quite intimidating. Maybe that is why I have always gone out of my way to make conversation with strangers when they are alone and look like they feel out of place, because I know what it feels like to be singled out and ignored. It's a pretty crappy feeling. But for some crazy reason, I was more determined than ever to accept this challenge and I knew this was the place that could offer me the education I was looking for. There were only about thirty spots open for the incoming class, and there were a lot more than thirty kids taking the exam that morning. Feeling so out of place made me question my ability, and I didn't think I had a chance of getting accepted. All of these kids had to be smarter than me. At least they looked a lot smarter—whatever that meant.

As I said, it was the longest exam I had ever taken in my life. I was so nervous that when I read the part that said "date of birth," I thought they wanted to know what day of the week I was born on. I raised my hand and told the proctor I didn't know what day I was born on. He must have thought I was a complete idiot. He asked me when my birthday was. I told him May 19th. He told me that I just needed to write my actual birthdate down, not the day. I couldn't have been more embarrassed. It took several minutes for me to regain my composure and actually start the exam after he walked away. I don't remember how long I sat there, but it seemed like forever. I finally focused on the questions and finished the test—convinced I had failed.

While my mother waited for me to take the test, she hung out with the other parents. Many families moved their homes to live closer to the school because they knew it was the best education in town. Others were frustrated that their children had failed the test before and were taking it for a second or third time. I don't think she realized what a big deal this place was until she hung out with the other grownups and waited for me to finish. When she told me about all of the conversations she overheard and participated in, I knew I was screwed.

It took a few weeks to get the results. I was pretty certain they would tell me that I didn't do well enough to join the incoming class. I was wrong. There were three girls and twenty-four boys that were asked to join the fifth-grade class that year, and I was one of them. I couldn't believe it! It was a very humbling moment for me. I actually did it. It was an important lesson for me; you don't know if you're capable of succeeding unless you try. I tried, and I did it. I felt really proud.

The town I lived in was roughly a one-hour commute from this new school. There were no buses that transported students from our town to the school, so my parents were forced to drive me. Fortunately, there were two other students from our community going there, so we were able to commute with their families. The school days were a lot longer than the public school I had been going to, which took some getting used to. Furthermore, all students were required to stay after school ninety minutes every day for either a sport or dance. The days were long, and the work was hard, but I was proud to be a part of it all.

The transition to a private school was a lot harder than I thought it would be, however. When I look back at my experience, I'm impressed with how resilient I was. I didn't fit in. I was an outcast from day one, yet I made the conscientious decision to suck it up and persevere. For starters, everything about my appearance was off. I didn't wear the right clothes or even the right shoes. My mom bought me the appropriate clothing, but I still didn't look like the other girls. I didn't have one-length hair that I wore in a ponytail with a ribbon that matched my clothes or my shoes. I knew the other students wore expensive clothing, but I remember thinking a lot of their outfits were ugly. Besides,

I didn't want to look like everyone else. My mom had gotten me three skirts that were cute and preppy, and I was happy with the new outfits she got me. I guess I was strong-willed from day one since I didn't want to do everything that was necessary to "fit in." My independent attitude didn't help with my assimilation to this new environment one bit.

I didn't know it would matter, but I soon discovered that my parents' profession also set me apart. My dad wasn't a doctor. My mom wasn't a lawyer. For some reason, selling insurance and real estate wasn't prestigious enough for my fellow students. I was looked down upon because of what my parents did for a living. It was pretty fucked up. They paid the same tuition as everyone else, so why did it matter? I had no idea then if my parents had a little or a lot of money. I had a great family, and I never equated wealth with the goodness of a person or as a measure of happiness. All I knew was that we traveled a lot, and I never wanted anything, so I knew we weren't poor. I was happy, well taken care of, and able to afford this place. I didn't know why that wasn't enough. Surprisingly, wealth mattered to my classmates more than it could have ever mattered to me. Believe me, I enjoy making a good living, but it doesn't mean anything if I'm not happy.

With regard to Fibromyalgia, I think it's important to try to pinpoint when your pain started so you can try to understand what triggered your symptoms. This is something I *really* want you to do, because you'll need that information to help you heal. Try to remember what was going on in your life when the pain started. You may or may not be surprised that there was a physical, emotional, or psychological event that acted as a catalyst to the onset of your condition.

There are many random events that stick in my mind that I'm sure led to many of my health issues. For example, other students would correct my vernacular, which was the most humiliating thing ever. I remember that happening like it was yesterday. I didn't know that I was expected to speak properly at all times, even when we were just hanging out in the lunchroom. I thought I could be myself with my peers, but I continually found myself struggling to fit in. Most of my peers were very proper and obviously had private schooling prior to attending this particular school. By their reaction to me, you'd think I was a damn hillbilly (I did have a pair of blue jean overalls that I really liked wearing). Yes, I said the word "ain't" occasionally. That didn't make me eligible to ride the short bus, for Christ's sake. But I was judged by it, and it sucked. I can't explain how embarrassing it is to have another student correct you when you are talking—especially at twelve years old.

There was no mistaking how different I was from the other kids from the very first day. For example, I didn't have aspirations of going to an Ivy League college, at least not in the fifth grade. To be honest, I wasn't even sure what an Ivy League college was. I knew that I wanted to go to college, but I didn't have an innate prejudice about what college I should or should not attend. It was obvious that many of my classmates had been programmed to believe they needed to pursue a certain path in life, regardless of how they felt about it. I didn't care about the status that accompanied one college over another until it was shoved down my throat for eight years.

The idea of prestige was an unfamiliar concept to me. I wanted to be successful and make a good living, but it wasn't the status or fame I aspired to, it was the reward of hard work and finding the path that made me happy and successful. I heard more from my parents about "if you want something, you must work for it." My mom also said more times than I count, "If you can't say something nice, don't say anything at all." Those were the types of values that were being ingrained in me, and I'm still proud of them. Achieving financial success was a definite bonus, but, at the end of the day, money doesn't buy happiness. It also doesn't buy good health or time.

All I knew is that I just wanted a better education so I could go to a better college and have more choices in life. Wasn't that good enough? I always knew that I wanted to find a career that I loved and, in return, make a good living. I didn't get the memo that said only certain aspirations were acceptable. Silly me.

I remember a time when a teacher asked us what we wanted to do for a living. This is another memory that had a tremendous impact on me—and not in a good way. One student said he wanted to be an anesthesiologist. I wasn't even sure what that was and I sure as heck didn't want to try to spell it. What fifth grader says they want to be an anesthesiologist? I had no idea. I assumed his mother or father must have hypnotized him when he was sleeping because what twelve-year-old aspires to put people to sleep for a living? Even back then, I had a sassy sense of humor. It was a shame that no one seemed to appreciate it. And to make matters worse, I decided to provide a smart-ass response with regard to my aspirations as an adult. I told the teacher that I wanted to drive a huge semi-truck across the country when I finished school. My truck would carry licorice and chocolate candy bars across the United States. It sounded liberating and adventurous. Believe me, my answer went over like a ton of bricks. And apparently, the bricks were attached to my feet because I was sinking fast.

I remember how the other students mocked me when I told them my plan. Homemade licorice and the chocolate candy bars called Choco'Lite were my favorite sugary obsessions, and those were the items I planned to transport across the country. I was pretty young at the time this discussion took place and the thought of traveling in a big truck really did sound appealing. Hell, I could have owned the trucking company and made stupid money for all they knew. It just wasn't a normal or acceptable career path. Okay, so maybe I wasn't normal. No one agreed with me that it was a sound occupational goal. I should have thrown in the towel that day. By all the standards at this elite school, I was a misfit.

It wasn't long until the teachers decided that I had a comprehension problem since I was having a hard time with the abundance of schoolwork we were expected to finish daily. I was only getting average grades on tests, which was a serious cause of concern to the powers that be.

Ultimately, I was forced to go into remediation. It was tedious and degrading as hell. There were only two of us who were set apart and forced to read short stories and answer questions until the words became a blur. I dreaded going to the room at the end of the hall on the left side of the second floor with the teacher who made me feel like I didn't belong at this school because, intellectually, there was something wrong with me. He made me feel dumb, or maybe that was my perception, but the feeling has stayed with me for the past forty-five years. I was embarrassed to be in remediation and I'm pretty sure the other kid felt the same way. We were the dummies who needed "extra help" while everyone else went to study hall.

I was having a hard time socially as well as academically and it made me want to be sick sometimes so I could avoid certain circumstances. It was such a bizarre time in my life, because I didn't belong, but I wasn't willing to quit either. I was determined to prove myself regardless of how I was treated. Now I can see that the way I was treated was a form of bullying, which no one talked about at the time. I just put myself into first-class survival mode and hunkered through.

I think I've spent my entire life welcoming challenges. I most definitely have my parents to thank for my perseverance and fortitude. Due to their constant encouragement and support, I was a fighter and a survivor. In retrospect, that has helped me in every aspect of my life. It was my choice to go to this school, and I knew it would offer me more opportunities in life. I was willing to make sacrifices to get a better education, and I didn't want to disappoint my parents by quitting. I think leaving the school would have been damaging to me as well in many ways. The crazy thing is that I never knew the sacrifices would make me sick.

CHAPTER 3

THE FIRST SYMPTOMS

I remember complaining that I had a lot of headaches when I started at this school. Sometimes they would get so bad that I would feel sick to my stomach or dizzy in the head. The first course of action was to take me to an eye doctor. The ophthalmologist said my eyes were basically fine, and that the headaches were probably caused by the dramatic increase in reading that was expected at my new school. He gave me a pair of reading glasses, even though he said my eyes were fine, and it didn't appear as if I really needed them. I imagine he was trying to appease me, so I went along with it. The glasses were supposed to keep my eyes from straining. I'm not sure they did much. They were probably just a slight magnification to give my eyes a little break. It was a long time ago, so it's hard to remember the specifics. All I clearly remember is that even when I wore the glasses, I still had headaches. That eye doctor was one of the first unproductive physicians that I saw.

Then I started getting a lot of stomach aches. I had a good diet and got regular exercise, but I was nervous a lot. I went to my doctor, and he said that all my stomach pain was due to ulcers caused by my nerves. I can't remember what the remedy was for that. I think it may have been taking Pepto-Bismol. He scared me though. He told me I'd get holes in my stomach that could never be repaired if I didn't get my nerves under control. While he may have said more to my mom, I didn't know. I only knew what stuck in my head. My nervousness was burning holes in my body, and I was screwed if I didn't get some control over my anxiety. My imagination has always been vivid, and the idea of permanent holes embedded in my stomach was a scary prospect. Apparently, my inability to deal with all the stressors of the new school was making me sick. Basically, it was my fault. My lack of coping skills in middle school was leading to holes in my gut. Big, massive craters that would probably kill me one day were what this young girl was envisioning. This kind of information made me even *more* stressed out. Yep, I was being weak even though I was doing everything in my power to be strong. Remember, at this point, I was thirteen years old. I was surrounded by teachers and advisors who expected us to act like adults or at least to perform like superhuman little grown-ups. Yes, it was stressful.

I probably should have been more honest with my parents about how difficult it was at school, but I didn't want to disappoint them. One of my sisters used to give them some trouble growing up and I never wanted to make waves or cause them any worry. I didn't like confrontation and I wanted my relationship with my parents to always be a positive one. I was the youngest of four and I always wanted to make them proud. Going to a private school was an incredible opportunity, and I was determined to make the best of it. Besides, the school was expensive, and I didn't want them to think they were wasting their money. And to be totally honest, I was embarrassed that I didn't fit in better. There was a part of me that believed I was a strong, bright young lady who should have been able to handle all the stressors of this private institution and assimilate into this new environment better. I was determined to prove myself. So, I put my best foot forward and continued to persevere.

I clearly remember feeling sick a lot. Having headaches and stomachaches on a daily basis will do that to a girl. Although my parents were sympathetic, they were also old school. You got up and did your job, no matter how you felt. And at that time in my life, my job was school. It's a work ethic that I wish more people had nowadays. It's commendable to get up every day and do your job to the best of your ability. I don't find anything admirable about calling in sick because you're feeling lazy or doing a half-ass job. I respect hard workers and have always considered myself one of them.

It's not that my parents didn't sympathize or love me. They dismissed a lot of my complaints because we were a family that focused on being positive and productive, not whiny and complacent. It should have made me upset, but it didn't. I knew they loved me. They were hard-working people who refused to let me succumb to a few minor aches and pains. Their fortitude was a blessing.

Middle school lasted from the fifth to the seventh grade. I had my ups and downs physically, but I made it through. I know that I felt lousy a lot of the time, but I was so busy that it was easy to set my ailments on a shelf and focus on other things.

Not only were the school days long, but as I previously mentioned, they expected each student to participate in sports after school when the academic day ended. Additionally, the girls were expected to take dance classes twice a week; specifically, ballet. Although I had never danced before, it quickly became clear that I was pretty good at it. Before long, I was able to get excused from sports so I could dance five days a week after school.

I loved ballet. It made me extremely happy. Unfortunately, it also brought me a lot of anguish. Unlike soccer or field hockey, ballet is a solitary sport. There wasn't the camaraderie that you get from belonging to an athletic team. It was also another thing that set me apart. It was worth it, though. I hated field hockey. I was once hit in the shins with a hockey stick and was immediately over it. I thought the whole concept of competitive sports where you had the potential of getting hurt was a little screwy. I begged the administration to excuse me from all sports so I could focus on ballet. They had never had a request like that before but were very supportive. For that, I was thankful. Bruises, dirt, sweat, blood… yeah, contact sports were not my thing. Walking around on my toes and twirling around in circles, now that was amazing, and it brought me a lot of joy.

During seventh grade, I was experiencing a lot of knee pain. At the end of the school year, I went to a doctor who diagnosed me with a condition called chondromalacia. He told me I needed to sit in a wheelchair and rest my knee for a couple of months so it could heal. There was no discussion about physical therapy or surgery, just rest. He gave me a shot of cortisone (which was excruciating), ordered a wheelchair, and sent me on my way. I remember that the needle that housed the cortisone was a gazillion inches long, and the solution was as thick as sludge. It took forever for the doctor to inject it into my body. I had an awful numb and restless sensation in my leg for seventy-two hours after he gave me the injection, and then all of the pain came back. Cortisone was not my friend. In fact, I had cortisone injections many years later and still had a lousy reaction to it and no relief. It was a futile attempt to make me better.

Our high school consisted of students from the eighth grade to the twelfth. I missed the beginning of high school because the buildings didn't have elevators and I was supposed to stay off my knee while it healed. That was such a strange and horrible time in my life. They didn't suggest crutches, which I could have used since it was only my left knee. I wasn't even allowed to start high school with everyone else. Once again, I was set apart from the masses. Isolation, as it turns out, makes you feel very alone. It can be a terrifying feeling.

After sitting around for several weeks, I was losing my mind. I was fairly friendly with a girl whose father was an orthopedic surgeon at the time for the Buffalo Bills. I went to him for a consultation to get a second opinion, because this sitting around thing was driving me bonkers. I should have gotten a second opinion from the beginning, but we didn't know any better.

Anyways, this sport's physician told me to get out of the chair and start weight training.

He instructed me to strengthen my quadriceps so that my muscles could support my weak knees. He also told me to stretch my calves for several minutes daily. His remedy was proactive, not passive. It was exactly what I needed and an important lesson for me to learn. From this point on, I knew I shouldn't rely on the opinion of one person since there could be a variety of ways of dealing with my problem—or any problem for that matter. That lesson has carried me through my multitude of ailments over the years. Ultimately, the decisions regarding my health should be mine. I've learned to listen to the advice from the various healthcare providers I've met over the years and come up with treatments that I am comfortable with. His attitude and approach to my knee condition were comforting and encouraging. I was so grateful for him. I wish I had met him before the doctor who shot me up with poison and told me to sit back and hope for the best.

Believe me, I haven't been complacent about my health care since that experience.

Fortunately, I was able to dance for another year, which I thoroughly loved. My dance teacher was from France. She was a short, feisty lady who liked to hit our various body parts with her stick in order to keep our postures in check. She was constantly telling us to keep our stomachs in, shoulders down, and po-po's (a.k.a. butts) tucked under. She saw a lot of potential in me and gave me leading roles. I enjoyed being on the stage and in the spotlight. It brought me a lot of joy. It also made me different. Not a surprise, huh?

Amidst all of these health problems was my real, hardcore introduction to being bullied. What happened during middle school was lame by comparison. When I was in the eighth grade, I developed a platonic relationship with my friend's brother, who was a senior at the time. Immediately, rumors started. He was very attentive, and I liked hanging out with him. He was a lot easier to talk to than the kids in my own grade. My experience with guys was extremely limited up to this point, and I didn't see why being friends with him was such a big deal. My sister Robin was six years older than me, and I remember hanging out with her and her friends and it was never an issue. This was a whole different story that changed my high school experience in some pretty shitty ways.

Certain things about our friendship stick out in my mind. For starters, he complimented me on how pretty I was. I vividly remember my friend being jealous because her brother thought I was cute. Sadly, I think she was probably one of the reasons all the nasty rumors started.

Jealousy can make people do hateful things. But I clearly remember thinking her jealousy was silly because she was a pretty girl too. And to be honest, the fact that he thought I was attractive didn't mean anything since he was a senior and I was in eighth grade. I was flattered, but that was it. Before long, my books and locker were desecrated with the words slut and whore. I also got rude and embarrassing prank phone calls on a regular basis on our home phone.

People accused me of sleeping with the brother. I admit there was a part of me that was attracted to him, but nothing ever happened; not even a kiss. In fact, I didn't have any sexual experience up to this point in my life aside from a few stolen kisses along the way. Having intercourse was not on my radar at that point by any stretch of the imagination. The thought of having sex was terrifying. I was only fourteen years old for Christ's sake! I most certainly wasn't mature enough to go all the way with anyone, especially a senior. At this point in my life, I never made it to second base, let alone any other of the bases. He was nice to me, which was a welcome surprise since most people treated me like crap and talked shit behind my back. I will admit that it was flattering to be liked by a senior. What girl wouldn't feel that way? We got along really well and could talk for hours. If he wanted any more than that, he didn't act on it. Unfortunately, once kids have pegged you as being a certain way, you're screwed. The torment went on for years. So did the pain.

The following year, I met a guy who I really liked. We were both in the ninth grade at the time. I admit that I pursued him pretty aggressively, and I'm glad I did. He was cute, smart, and athletic. Most of all, he wasn't as preppy as the other guys in our class, which was a welcome change. I liked the fact that he was different. He was a really good athlete and smart enough to get a full scholarship to the school. I was thrilled when he finally noticed me, and we started dating.

He never received ridicule like I did because he belonged to three athletic teams. He had friends outside of our relationship, which made all the difference in the world. Although we spent as much time together as possible, he was really good at sports and had friends on all the teams he belonged to. He was a popular guy, and I was honored to be his girlfriend. We ended up dating all through high school and even through our first year of college. He was the love of my life for almost five years, and I treasure the relationship I had with him. But even though he was well liked in the athletic community, we both had to suffer the jealous and petty attitudes of our classmates. I'll never understand why people can't just be accepting when a couple is happy together instead of throwing daggers, but I guess that is part of being a teenager. Once again, the jealous monsters reared their ugly heads our way. He was able to shrug off what other people said about us, but I wasn't that strong.

The boys in my grade gave me a hard time because I only dated one guy during our high school career. For the most part, I didn't care, because I knew

I was dating the best guy in the class. There was another part of me that prayed everyone would just accept him and me as a couple and not talk about us. Even though I was secure in my relationship, I had a really hard time dealing with when other boys would pick on me, as I just wasn't the type of girl who fought back. I didn't want to give anyone any ammunition to antagonize me.

I remember an incident when one of my classmates started a rumor that my family had been killed in an automobile accident. One night, I got a weird and scary prank phone call while my parents were out of town that my family had died in a car accident. There were no cell phones at the time, so it was more difficult to communicate with my family. My parents were due home that night, so there was no way for me to know if they really had been in an accident or not. I remember being so scared and crying continuously until they arrived home safely. When they got home, they couldn't understand why I was so upset and kind of blew off my theatrics because they knew nothing had happened, and, obviously, they were fine. What resonates the most with me is the terror I felt over the idea that my folks had died. It was an inexcusable prank that was very traumatic for me. Since then, I've learned that trauma can be detrimental to your health.

The next day I found out that other students had heard the rumor. Most of them thought I had been killed in the accident along with my family. All day, kids were looking at me like they had seen a ghost. It was a horrible, unforgivable prank, and it affected me in ways I can't explain. The fear of thinking my family had been killed was extremely traumatic. Thank God it was a hoax. But what kind of nutjob would even start a rumor like this? That is the kind of fear and terror that can really wreak havoc on your body—and it did.

A few of the girls in my class were jealous because I was the only one my boyfriend wanted to date. I never felt the need to apologize because he liked me, and we had a great thing going on, and neither of us had the desire to date anyone else. Although we were only teenagers, my boyfriend and I had a great relationship filled with joy and passion. We loved each other, plain and simple. It was very special. It was the kind of first love that people read in fairy tales.

Sadly, we didn't get much support from anyone else—including his parents.

Once his parents found out we were sexually active, they tried even harder to discourage our relationship. While it didn't work, it did make things much more stressful. I recall always being afraid of going to his house. His parents were not welcoming at all and treated me like a pariah. I always felt like they blamed me for being a distraction from their golden son's academic and athletic career. I remember an incident when his father chastised me for biting my nails. It was so embarrassing. Believe me, you would have bitten your nails too if you could have seen the way they treated me sometimes. It concerned him that nail biting was unhealthy and suggested that I was a very nervous girl. Yeah, I was nervous around them, which is why I gnawed on my nails like a starving rat. The truth is, all I wanted was for them to like me. After his father insulted me, I never bit my nails again.

No matter how much grief they gave us, we had a great relationship, and I didn't have any regrets. From early on, I believed in monogamy and treasured the experience I had with him. It was also good practice for the future. Committing to a guy was really important to me. It made me happy. That's probably why I've been married for nearly forty years.

The administration thought we were too demonstrative in public and brought my parents to the school for a conference with the principal. The school was concerned about the fact that my boyfriend and I held hands and outwardly showed affection (if they only knew what we did in some of the deserted hallways…). My parents were nonplussed. We were horny teenagers who were in love. They understood that and dismissed the school as being uptight. I was so relieved that they had my back. At least someone did. The administration mandated that I talk to the counselor at school. Apparently, being in a loving, happy relationship suggested some kind of mental abnormality that required professional help. The thought of therapy made me want to scream at them, but I conceded to keep the peace.

I recently asked my mom what she remembered about that meeting. She told me that the administration found it disconcerting that I saved a seat for my boyfriend at school assemblies. That sounds wicked naughty, doesn't it? They asked the principal if we were ever found doing something inappropriate. He said no. My mother remembers the whole discussion being a terrible waste of time and thinking they were being petty and ridiculous.

By the end of ninth grade, my knee was shot. It hurt all of the time and I was forced to quit ballet. It was a horrible time in my life. I was excused from dance, and participating in sports was not an option since I didn't like them and wasn't healthy enough to play anyways. I felt extreme jealousy when another girl became the lead in the dance productions. All I could think was that I should have been the lead, not her. The whole thing sucked. I became so distraught that it was a blessing that I was seeing a counselor at school. She was amazing, and I'm not sure I would have survived high school without her. Gail Mordaunt was my savior that year.

About a year after I quit ballet, I missed dancing, and I missed being active, so I joined an aerobic jazz class with my mom. The class was held in a church parking lot in a neighboring suburb. We had such a good time dancing and singing that it didn't even feel like a type of exercise, and it was low impact enough so that it didn't bother my knees. I decided that I wanted to develop an aerobic jazz program at my school, so I approached the administration about teaching aerobic classes as an alternative to sports or dance. By some crazy twist of fate, this stuffy institution said yes! By my junior year, I was given the permission I needed to start an aerobic dance class that took place every day after school for ninety minutes in a room above the hockey rink. I knew I wanted to make it harder than what I did in the church parking lot, but my goal was to make it fun. I loved music and I loved to dance, so this was my chance to do both. My knee still bugged me, but I didn't care. I was having a lot of fun, and it was easier on me than dancing in pointe shoes. By my senior year, my aerobics program became a varsity sport. I even had some of the teachers take my classes. It was one of the best experiences I had in high school because it was a lot of fun. To be honest, I enjoyed being in the spotlight and being in control. I was also proud that so many people joined my classes and had fun with me.

During this time, I still had random aches and pains, but I didn't care. I smoked a fair amount of pot, which helped with my physical and emotional pain. And, for the most part, I was happy. I was dating the cutest guy in my grade, having a blast teaching aerobics, and doing decently in school. The bullying had become subtler. There were incidents here and there, but I developed a pretty thick hide (or so I thought). I didn't have many friends, but I had a boyfriend, and he was all I felt I needed. I was friendly with many girls in the class, but I didn't hang out with them very often. Although I still felt like an outcast, I focused on the good things in my life. Complaining served no purpose. It still doesn't. Obviously, it was that one important lesson my parents instilled in me that carried me through my developmental years.

Even to this day, I have very few female friends. I'm very committed to my husband and my children and put most of my energy into them. I feel selfish about sharing my time with others. I'm a lot like my mom that way. She was devoted to my dad for forty years and now to her boyfriend for over thirty. Sometimes I wish I had more women in my life, but I just don't think I'm wired that way because of the trauma I experienced with a variety of girls growing up. Besides, I've spent my career with women in the salon, and that has been more rewarding than words could ever express. The women I've worked with in my career have brought me joy and filled that female void, and I am extremely grateful for that. But at the end of the day, I just want to be with my husband and my kids.

When you go to a private school, there is a lot of pressure to go to the right college. When my mom and I met with my counselor to discuss my options, she tried to convince me to solely apply to all-women's colleges. I remember this conference like it happened yesterday. Both my mother and I laughed when she suggested that. She said that it was obvious I was obsessed with my boyfriend, and the best thing for me would be to go to a college with no men. Thank goodness my mother had my back on this issue as well. She told the counselor that she would never consider going to an all-women's college and wasn't going to encourage me to go to one either. My mom continued by saying that going to a single-sexed college was not real life, and she strongly believed that college should be a preparation for real life, not a segregated one. Since I was going to be interacting with men when I got a job, I should interact with them in college as well. The counselor did not appreciate our negative opinion about all-women's colleges and sported a pretty bad attitude when we scoffed at her suggestion. Apparently, she went to an all-women's college and thought they were the "cat's meow"—as my father used to say. Let's just say that my mom and I basically hissed at her. That was the end of that meeting. I was forced to find a college on my own.

I randomly picked five colleges out of a large book. I was accepted by two and rejected by the other three. If I did my homework, I would have realized that my SAT scores weren't even remotely good enough for the places I applied to. Sadly, since I had no help finding a place to go, I tried getting into schools that were way above my credentials. Oh well. Live and learn.

Leaving my boyfriend and going our separate ways for college was heartbreaking. Saying goodbye to him was one of the hardest things I had ever done in my life up to that point. I cried for days. My parents were worried about me. My grief consumed me, and everything hurt, including my heart. I went to Lynchburg (in Virginia), and he went to Hamilton (in New York). It was a long-distance relationship that was very difficult to maintain, especially since we had no way of communicating while we were at school. The year was 1983. There were no such things as cell phones or the Internet. I had a pay phone at the end of my hall. Needless to say the long-distance relationship scenario was the start of the end for us.

College was more challenging than I thought it would be, and it had nothing to do with academics. As it turned out, I found the schoolwork relatively easy. It was the other stuff that I had problems with. I didn't realize what an independent thinker I was until I was submerged into this conservative Baptist community in the beautiful mountains of Lynchburg, Virginia. I had a strong Northern personality that didn't quite fit in (big surprise). I was open-minded and strong-willed, and I had difficulty accepting the Southern mentality.

The school I went to was far more restrictive for women than men. For example, the guys could have kegs of beer in their dorm rooms any night of the week, while the ladies could not. Fed up with this, I bought a keg and hid it in my shower. Believe it or not, I almost got kicked out of the school because of this. Apparently, I violated a rule about having no alcohol in our dorms, even though no staff ever saw the keg. What century was I living in? I got fined and put on probation even though they never had physical proof that I had done anything wrong. Yes, I purchased a keg and hid it in a shower, but the guys had kegs all the time right in the open and no one said anything! It was then that I realized that this was not the place for me. My liberal, Northern mindset would not allow me to be treated like this.

The people I met at school were also prejudiced against other religions and other races, which I didn't understand at all. It was the most backward environment and way of thinking that I was ever exposed to. I didn't agree with their philosophy one bit, and I realized pretty quickly that I needed to transfer to a school in the Northern part of our country.

My freshman year of college was when the night terrors began. At eighteen years old, I developed a childhood affliction that is uncommon in adults. I would wake up in the middle of the night screaming like I was being brutally attacked. It scared the shit out of my roommate, and it terrified me too. It was the same nightmare every time. A dark creature held me down, and I was powerless. It was awful. Whenever I had a night terror, the following day I would feel achy and exhausted. It was as if my body was affected systemically by the fear that consumed my brain while I was sleeping. It was a creepy feeling that was hard to explain. It made me afraid to sleep. To this day, I still have trouble sleeping, and I still have night terrors occasionally. It has been a difficult affliction that has plagued me for far too long.

Lynchburg wasn't the right fit for me. I wasn't happy. I gained a lot of weight in a very short amount of time. It was the first time in my entire life I was heavy, and I was very embarrassed by what I looked like and what I felt like. Most girls gain the freshman fifteen; I gained the freshman forty… the first semester. Happiness has a lot to do with how you feel. I wasn't happy so I felt like shit, which caused me to feel like I looked even worse.

I did make one friend that year, and we are still close friends today. Cindy was the only shining light on what was becoming my very dark existence. One day, she walked into my dorm room to say hi and I told her I didn't want any friends. I was pretty grumpy by this point. She told me she felt the same way. We were both miserable at Lynchburg, had put on a lot of weight since school began, and had spent a lot of time alone. It was our commiserating that brought us together. She was the only thing I am thankful for that happened that year. Her friendship got me through my freshman year; I will always be grateful for her, and I still treasure our relationship today.

One night Cindy and I decided to find a place where we could go dancing. It was the events that followed that night that solidified my need to get out of Lynchburg.

That night, I met and quickly became friends with a Black bodybuilder Cindy and I met at the dance club. He was a really nice guy and a lot of fun to hang out with. More importantly, he was sexy as hell on the dance floor. Normally I wouldn't mention the color of his skin, but it was a significant part of this memory. We both loved dancing, and it was fun for my girlfriend and I to have someone to go dancing with. At the time, I didn't realize how racist of a community I was living in. I was already frustrated with the double standard at the college, but I didn't experience such outward racism until I met this guy. I expected a more liberal mindset in college, but I found out quickly that befriending a Black man was going to be my kiss of death amongst my peers. As soon as I brought him to our dorm, the other girls in the hall called me a "n*****" lover" and completely ostracized me. I had never encountered this kind of blatant prejudice before. It was horrible and it made me sad. It also pissed me off. I think I kept the friendship alive in part because he scared many of my classmates, and our friendship made them uncomfortable. To be honest, I wanted them to feel uncomfortable. He was just a person, like any of us. He just had a darker complexion. I didn't get it. It was funny because I never really made a distinction one way or the other about the color of a person's skin. Suddenly I was surrounded by people who made that difference a really big deal. I briefly felt the hatred that this guy felt every day of his life. It was so unfair.

The community as a whole did not approve of a relationship between a Black man and a white woman. I remember going out to Sunday brunch one time and a family next to us turned their children's chairs away from our table so they couldn't see us sitting together. It was blatant and rude. As a white woman, I never felt that kind of prejudice before, and it frightened me. It was horrible to be judged by my friend's skin color. I didn't understand why any Black person would want to live in this ignorant town. I knew I couldn't stay there with such narrow-minded people.

This kind of negativity was really difficult for me to deal with. I found myself feeling more exhausted and achier daily. I hung out in my room a lot because I wasn't treated the same way anymore, and I was becoming depressed. There was a local restaurant that would deliver submarine sandwiches and beer to my dorm room. I loved that place. Sadly, it added to my weight gain and made it even easier to hibernate in my room. I hid as much as possible because I began to seriously resent the community I was living in. I went from being well-liked to being a pariah. In addition, the more I lay around, the bigger I got and the crappier I felt. It was an ugly, vicious cycle that I didn't think I'd ever break.

I decided to kick ass academically so I could transfer to anywhere I wanted to. And that's exactly what I did. I transferred to the University of Rochester in Rochester, New York, since I knew that I had a more Northern mentality and would never survive living down South. Focusing on a new school and a new city was a positive step to my mental and hopefully physical health.

I learned a lot more than academics at Lynchburg. I experienced a rude awakening to racial prejudice and being around such hatred and negativity made me emotionally and physically ill. That experience reinforced my belief that I should always be an accepting kind of person who doesn't judge others. It was ugly and hurtful, and I couldn't and still can't understand how people can treat others with such hatred and disdain. I vowed to remain open-minded to all people because that small glimpse of prejudice opened my eyes to a whole other world that frightened and bewildered me.

Leaving Lynchburg was a wonderful feeling. It felt liberating to head back to New York.

I had no regrets and was so relieved that I'd never have to go back there again.

CHAPTER 4

MY FAVORITE OLD GUY

I was extremely relieved when my first year of college was over. Having a more content state of mind always helps with the way you feel physically and emotionally. During the summer between my freshman and sophomore year, I secured a full-time job at my father's insurance business, and I enjoyed being home. Some unfortunate things occurred between my boyfriend and me that summer, which ultimately led to the demise of our relationship. After nearly five years together, the loss was monumental. It was hard for me to separate the way my body felt when I was sad. At the time, I didn't put two and two together, but looking back I realized that the sadness definitely intensified my physical pain.

During that summer, I was the victim of a sexual assault. It was an incident that I only recently admitted to because I found a therapist who enabled me to admit it out loud, accept that it wasn't my fault and ultimately put it to rest. It was the kind of trauma that I buried deep down inside of me because it was ugly, and I'm the kind of person who doesn't like to dwell on the bad shit. Unfortunately, burying it wasn't the healthiest way to deal with it, but it was the only way I knew to make it go away—or so I thought. But I refuse to beat myself up about the way I didn't handle it either. I was a victim, and it's never too late to deal with your demons. Now, I can move on. I'm convinced that the experience scarred me in more ways than I can put into words, and I know that it intensified my nightmares. Since I recently brought the memory back to my conscious brain, I can finally put it to rest. Suffice to say, all trauma is bad, whether it is physical, psychological, sexual, or emotional.

As I was dealing with the breakup of my high school sweetheart, my eighty-seven-year-old grandfather fell and broke his hip. He had surgery, but there were complications. He was in the hospital when I was getting ready to transfer to the University of Rochester. It was so hard saying goodbye to him. He had been my next-door neighbor and traveling companion for the previous seven years, and I loved him with all my heart. When I was saying goodbye to him, I couldn't stop crying. He was the first loved one that I was close to that was going to die, and it really frightened me. He was a very religious man and believed in Heaven. I remember like it was yesterday when he scolded me for crying. He told me he was ready to die and there was no reason for me to be sad. That was a really hard thing to hear, and no matter what he said, I couldn't stop crying. I was grief-stricken.

The day I said my final goodbye to him, he told me that my grandma was going to yell at him when he got to heaven for growing a beard, since she forbade him to grow one while they were married. That made me feel a little better. He had a strong faith and was ready to move on. I understood that it was selfish of me to be so sad, because he was at peace with it. Even though it was an important lesson about life and death, it was a difficult time.

I transferred to Rochester with a very heavy heart, because I wasn't sure if I'd ever see my grandfather again. The school didn't have housing for me, so I was forced to live in a seedy motel for the first month. There were rooms that were rented by the hour and the neighborhood was sketchy and unsafe. I had to pass through a low-income housing project to get to the motel and I never felt safe traveling through the area at night. The whole setup was extremely inappropriate for a single, nineteen-year-old woman. There were five other students living there at the same time. Within my first week of staying there, all of their rooms got broken into. I got lucky because my room was at the end of the corridor facing the street. After three weeks of living there, there was a shooting on the premises. That was the last straw; I moved out the following month.

I was scared living in the motel that month and I knew I had to find a way out of there. I transferred to a new school where I knew virtually no one (again), which wasn't easy. I was living in a dangerous place. My grandpa was dying. I wasn't dating anyone. I felt very alone. It was a frightening time. Since then, I have realized that fear can wreak some serious havoc on your body, especially when it is ongoing. Over the years, whenever I have felt scared, my body physically hurts. It's difficult to explain, but it is what happens to me. It is as real as the words on this page. I seem to have a physiological response to fear. My body doesn't like it and neither do I. That's probably why I don't watch scary movies; I don't like to be frightened. It hurts too much.

When my mom called me to tell me that my grandfather died, I was devastated. Even though I cognitively knew it was going to happen, it was still a shock when it did. The funeral was sad. Up to this point in my life, I had never seen my dad cry. He cried that day. He loved my grandfather very much. My father was a strong, happy guy who dealt with things strategically and with humor. Not this day. He was so sad; it made the day that much harder.

After the funeral, I went back to school. I found a new place to live, a job teaching aerobics, and I started dating. I tried to keep as busy as possible. I learned from the get-go that being busy was the best medicine when I was feeling lousy. It was a good distraction. Moping around never helped. Being productive was pivotal to achieving success in life. It was that all-important lesson my folks taught me that kept me focused and determined.

Shortly after my grandpa died, I met Mark. That was in October of 1984. There is a part of me that is convinced my grandfather had something to do with us getting together. He came into my life when I needed someone desperately. Before him, I went on a handful of first dates with guys that were pretty or had hot bodies but were either dull, arrogant, or just plain yucky. Mark was a breath of fresh air. He was ambitious and feisty and like no one I had ever met. I knew a relationship with him could be a fun challenge. I was right. He was bright, unpredictable, and loyal to a fault. It looked like I finally met an interesting man. As it turns out, he is still in my life; we've been together since the fall of 1984.

During that year, I had a lot of lower abdominal issues. My regular doctor sent me to a gynecologist since the issues didn't seem GI related. The gynecologist thought I had a condition called pelvic inflammatory disease, which would make it probable that I would never have children. It was so frightening to think I wouldn't be able to have a family since I was only nineteen at the time and knew I'd want kids one day. The doctor suggested I have exploratory surgery to figure out what was going on inside of my body.

The surgery was inconclusive. Gee, what a surprise. At nineteen, I wasn't sure if I could ever have kids, but the doctor didn't really know one way or the other. I had recurrent, crippling lower abdominal pain that no one could find an answer for. Nothing with my health was ever easy. What I didn't know at the time was that I was going to have many more years of doctors giving me inconclusive diagnoses. Actually, it would be decades. He did suggest that I might have pulled my abdominal muscles working out. If that were the case, then I needed to be patient because it would take some time to heal. I was so angry that I went through an exploratory surgery that was inconclusive and probably completely unnecessary. I spent the next month resting from any physical activity in case it was a muscle issue. I took a break from teaching aerobics and working out. Over the next few weeks, my stomach felt better. It must have been strained muscles. I felt frustrated, relieved, and a whole slew of other emotions that are difficult to put into words.

I still had intense pain with intercourse, however, so I decided to find a local gynecologist to see what he thought of my stomach issues. During my initial exam, he felt my entire abdominal area. He casually asked me when the last time I had a bowel movement was. I couldn't remember. It had probably been at least a week before this appointment. He laughed and said he absolutely didn't think I had pelvic inflammatory disease. On the contrary, he told me I needed to learn how to go to the bathroom on a regular basis. Apparently, my small intestine was so full that it was pressing against my vaginal wall. My lady parts were fine. I just needed to take a serious shit. When I look back at that time in retrospect, I remember feeling very flu-ish back then as well. I think that the perpetual constipated state I was living in was poisoning my fragile system. Even today, over thirty years later, I experience a direct correlation between irregularity and achiness. When I'm not regular, I'm in more pain. My body is very sensitive to any irregularities, and it doesn't like being full of shit—literally or figuratively. It can be very annoying. Regular elimination is more important than most people realize. If you're full of shit, it's really not a good thing.

He recommended that I examine my diet and take stool softeners on a regular basis until I got my bowels working properly again. I hadn't been regular since I started college and put on my "freshman forty" weight gain. I forgot how much better I felt when I went to the bathroom on a daily basis. Once I had that under control, my vaginal pain disappeared. This is another circumstance where I should have considered getting a second opinion before the surgery.

I knew I had to make a change. I was overweight, constipated, tired, and pretty unhappy with my body, which totally affected my emotional and psychological state. I decided that the first step was to remove all fast food and beer from my diet. I lost twenty-five pounds in less than two months. I read somewhere that the average American has fifteen pounds of waste in their body. I think I definitely had more than a few pounds setting up residency in my colon. Once I changed my diet, I began to feel human again. I didn't realize how much fast food I consumed on a weekly basis. There was definitely a correlation between how I ate and how I felt. It just took me a long time to figure it out.

This was the point in my life when I started being more cognizant of my diet. It didn't take long for me to realize that some foods made me feel especially lousy. I didn't necessarily remove the aggravating foods from my diet, however. I just knew that if I ate fast food, I'd feel gassy, achy, and bloated. That doesn't mean I avoided those foods; I just accepted the fact that they'd make me feel crappy. Eating properly and "clean" as it's referred to these days isn't as easy as it seems, but it is crucial for the way my body feels.

I experienced a lot of changes that year. I changed schools, moved to a new city, lost my grandpa, and fell in love. Whether a change is good or bad in your life, it has the ability to affect how you feel. I am sensitive to all changes that occur in my life no matter if they are positive or negative. Obviously, the negative ones are more detrimental to my health, and that has been an interesting lesson for me to learn.

CHAPTER 5

THE ACCIDENT FROM HELL

Life went on, and I felt better about things. Mark and I fell in love and got married. I still had random aches and pains, but I was able to ignore them for the most part. I kept busy. I went to graduate school and held down two jobs. Overall, my body was feeling okay. Sadly, things didn't remain okay. On April 26, 1990, I got a call from my brother very early one morning. He told me our dad was electrocuted putting his sailboat away in Florida. He was only sixty years old and in a coma. It was very serious, and he was in critical condition. I was really scared.

Mark and I had just been on vacation with my parents. We left the Florida Keys on a Tuesday, and the accident happened the next day. Although his heart stopped and his breathing seized, two men at the scene of the accident managed to bring him back to life with CPR. He had to be airlifted to a hospital in Miami since the local hospital in the Florida Keys didn't take severe trauma cases. His body was severely burned from the electricity, and he was in a coma for a month. The neurologist in Florida told us to pray he never woke up, because his neurological damage was too extensive, and his brain was fried. After a month passed, my mom had him flown to Buffalo, NY, so he could be near our family. When he woke up, his brain was indeed fried. Turns out the neurologist was right. It was the kind of nightmare you wouldn't wish on anyone.

Sadly, his brain could have never survived the excessive trauma. It is a long, sad story that is still difficult for me to even talk about without tearing up. Ultimately, his brain injury was too severe for there to be any hope of recovery. On the other hand, he had a strong body that wasn't ready to die. It took one and a half years for him to finally pass.

While he was in the hospital, Mark and I decided to start a family. I had this intense need to continue that whole circle-of-life concept, and I felt blessed that my husband was on board with my desire to have a baby. It was actually a funny conversation that I love to share. Mark was perming my hair (he's a hairdresser, and perms were still pretty popular back then) and I informed him, while he was wrapping the back of my head with perm rods, that I ran out of birth control pills. That ingenious gynecologist I found back when I was nineteen years old who confirmed I didn't have PID always provided me with my pills for free. He only had a few packs left when I last visited him, so he told me to call him when I got low again. When I told Mark I was out of pills, he told me to call the doctor and ask for some more. I told him I didn't want to. Curious, he asked me if I wanted to have a baby. I told him that the running out of pills and Dad in the hospital were a sign. That was the end of the discussion. We were going to try to have a baby. Since my father had been transferred to a hospital in Buffalo from one in Miami, it was possible for Mark and me to visit him every weekend. Every Saturday after work, we would visit my dad in the hospital, and then spend the rest of the weekend with my mom. She was married to my father for forty years and kept vigil by his side. My heart bled for her. Since they worked side by side in their privately owned business, they were together all of the time. Since my parents spent so much time together, the void was excruciating for my mother.

My mom and dad were incredible role models. They had a very happy marriage and a strong business partnership. That made the accident even more tragic. I hated the thought of her being alone. Fortunately, Mark was adamant that we both go to Buffalo every weekend to stay with her. He didn't want her to be alone either. His compassion for my mom made me love him even more. In fact, his support and love for my family during this whole nightmare solidified the fact that he was the best man to have in my corner in difficult times. He still is.

I'm pretty confident I got pregnant at my parents' house during one of those weekends we were staying with my mom. I had a dream that night after we had been intimate that we were going to be blessed with a son. That dream became a reality.

The pregnancy was hard. I had morning sickness that lasted twenty-four seven for the first four months. I had inexplicable pains in my hips, legs, and back. It didn't help that I cried all the time. My dad had no idea who any of us were and he was withering away in a damn hospital, which was unbearable to witness. It was a horrible time in all of our lives. Although he looked like my dad, he wasn't there anymore. He swore, yelled, moaned, and rambled nonsense. The whole thing sucked more than I could ever put into words. Brain injuries are a nightmare. We tried to have hope, even though the doctors told us that it would be impossible for him to recover. On the one hand, it was really difficult letting him go but on the other hand, it was impossible watching him suffer.

During the pregnancy, my gynecologist suggested that I get a flu shot. I had never had one before, but he told me it would protect my baby. I couldn't argue with that. It never occurred to me that I should question whether or not the shot could have any adverse reactions to me. All I knew was if it would protect my baby then I was in. My pregnancy continued to be difficult, but I had too much going on in my life to analyze what was going on with me. It was all about the baby and my dad.

The call saying that he finally passed put me into labor. I was thirty-nine weeks along, so it was a safe time to have the baby. It was a long and extremely arduous labor because my body wasn't completely ready to deliver. My doctor said the stress put me into emotional labor and although it could take a long time to deliver this baby, it was going to happen sooner than later. Twenty-six hours after the first contraction, I successfully delivered a baby boy, who we named Adryan Robert.

Our son was born the day after my dad died. I can hear "Circle of Life" by Elton John playing in my head as I'm writing this. We used my father's name as our son's middle name. It was much too close to name him Robert. When I was released from the hospital, we drove directly to my father's memorial service.

Memories from that weekend are sketchy in my brain. There were too many emotions happening all at once. I was happy about the baby, sad about my dad, exhausted from the delivery, and all of the emotions… It was just overwhelming. All I do know is that I got my circle-of-life experience. It was heartbreaking and miraculous all in one.

Between the stress and pain of my father's passing and the delivery, my body wasn't able to produce milk. I tried for two weeks to nurse our son, but it was futile. It's not surprising that I wasn't strong or healthy enough to feed my baby considering the events that transpired in our lives, but it was still difficult to deal with. Both of my sisters were feeding machines for their babies, while I barely had spit coming out of me. There was too much sadness to make it possible for me to feed my son. The pediatrician suggested we use formula, since I wasn't producing enough milk.

I know it isn't easy for every woman to breastfeed, but it made me feel incompetent. To make matters even worse, the switch to formula didn't go well either. The first formula caused him to projectile vomit numerous times. That was fun. The first time it happened, I swear the vomit flew six feet from where I was holding him. It was an exorcism of baby puke. It shouldn't surprise me that he had a sensitive stomach considering all the anguish I experienced while I was pregnant with him. In the end, we went through a half dozen formulas before we found one that he didn't spit back up on us. And it wasn't any of the expensive ones. It was Gerber Low Iron, and we got it from B.J.'s. It may seem like a small victory, but it was a Godsend at the time.

Before I knew it, I was pregnant again. The morning sickness was just as awful. Once again, my doctor suggested I get a flu shot since it is recommended to get one yearly. It never occurred to me not to get it. I got it to protect myself from getting the flu and, more importantly, to protect the baby. I was achy a lot but chalked it up to the pregnancy. The overall body pains were much worse this time around, and I was having a difficult time dealing with all of the pain and discomfort.

I taught aerobics through my first pregnancy, but I had to stop when I got pregnant the second time. The pain was just too intense. I tried acupuncture, massage, and physical therapy. None of them really helped but I was determined to find something that made me more comfortable. I had a brace made for me to support my hips because they hurt so badly. It didn't help. Pregnancy was not my friend. Our children were born healthy, but I was pretty miserable through the whole thing. It was worth it, but it sucked all the same.

When I was seven months pregnant with our second child, I experienced another traumatic event that was pretty horrific. While my dad was in the hospital dying, my siblings and I bought our mom a three-pound Maltese dog. He was the cutest puppy you'd ever want to meet. It was becoming difficult for my mother to take care of the dog since she spent so much time at work and with my dad in the nursing home, so Mark and I decided that we would adopt her dog so she didn't have to worry about him. Mom named him MR. GGs (which are the initials of my siblings and me). He went to work with us every day and was such a joy.

One day, I was walking down the street with the dog. I was going to pick up our son from Mark's parents, who lived around the corner from us and were babysitting him while we went out to dinner. MR. GGs was under two years old at the time and still weighed about three pounds. Because he was so small, we didn't put a collar on him because his neck was too fragile. At the time, it never occurred to me to buy a small harness so I could walk him on a leash. As I was walking around a bend in the road, I saw a man walking a large German shepherd towards me. I asked the man if the dog was friendly. He simply shrugged his shoulders in a non-committal manner. MR. GGs ran up to the dog wanting to say hi and play, and I could see the German shepherd wagging his tail. Before I knew what was happening, the shepherd picked up my dog in his mouth and started shaking it like a rag doll. I was afraid to get near the animal since I was pregnant, and the dog's owner did nothing but tell the dog (his name was Kilgore, by the way) to drop it. I really wanted to kick the animal, but I was too afraid he might bite me, so I couldn't risk it. There was no way I was jeopardizing the baby growing inside of me. As soon as I realized this guy was absolutely useless and wasn't going to do anything, I screamed my husband's name as loud as possible over and over again. Although I wasn't visible from our home, Mark heard me screaming and came running.

When Mark came running around the bend, he saw how Kilgore was crushing our dog.

He started to punch the dog as aggressively as possible, but the shepherd wouldn't let go of MR. GGs. When it was obvious Kilgore wouldn't let go, Mark pried the dog's mouth open with his hands and yelled for me to call for help. I ran next door to my in-laws to call 911 while a neighbor took Mark and the dog to the vet. While I was on the phone, my father-in-law walked into the kitchen. I yelled for him to find Mark. He took off without question. When I hung up the phone, I felt like I was going to faint. I walked outside and collapsed. I sat on my in-law's driveway in my short, white maternity dress with black polka-dots and flat black sandals trying to catch my breath. I was crying hysterically, hyperventilating, and having contractions. It was so scary. I was so afraid something bad was going to happen to the baby if I didn't calm down, but all I could hear was my dog crying and looking at me as the shepherd crushed his bones. I didn't even realize my father-in-law raced to the vet to be there for Mark; I just knew he went after him and that he would find him.

Mark returned with our dog in a box. He was covered in blood, our dog's and his own. A police officer and an ambulance arrived shortly after. The police officer ordered the owner of the shepherd to get proof that the dog was vaccinated. The man returned with his wife to my in-law's house. Ironically, the wife was nine months pregnant and actually due that day. The man asked Mark what the vet said. Mark was crying and said, "He said my dog was dead." The man said nothing further, no apologies or any words of condolence. He was an unsympathetic asshole. The wife approached the driveway and looked at me sitting on the pavement holding my stomach, crying and trying to catch my breath. She said nothing. It was surreal. The whole experience was a nightmare. Like it wasn't bad enough that their dog killed MR. GGs, they didn't have the decency to even apologize.

We ended up suing the family so they would be forced to euthanize the dog. Even though we had several neighbors give testimony that the owners mistreated the dog, and the dog was violent and neglected, it was the dog's first offense. The family was required to remove the dog from the neighborhood, but not to euthanize him. It was a small victory.

Fortunately, I didn't go into labor that day, but I was really traumatized by the experience. I had several nightmares and cried a lot after it happened. Since I was so preoccupied with my first child coming right after Dad died, I don't think I grieved properly over his passing. Watching the shepherd crush MR. GGs was the catalyst that released all my grief from my father's passing as well as the dog. I was heartbroken, and I felt like the tears would never end.

Although Mark was also grieving, he was my rock. He kept reminding me that it was only a dog and I had to take care of the baby and me. I think that was hard for him to say because he loved the dog as much as I did, but someone needed to stay strong, and it sure as hell wasn't going to be me. I was a wreck.

Our daughter Kaylah Dora arrived at thirty-nine weeks just like our son did. This time around, I was able to nurse her for six weeks, which made me happy. It wasn't as long as my sisters by any stretch of the imagination, but I was impressed. For once, my body was cooperating.

After the second child was born, I couldn't handle the pain in my hips. Even though I wasn't able to teach aerobics during the second pregnancy, I continued to exercise despite all the pain in my joints. It got to the point where I couldn't deal with how much everything hurt. It was also at this point that I felt compelled to see if there was something clinically wrong with my hips or low back. My doctor sent me to a popular orthopedic hip surgeon in our area. Because I continued to work out and stretch regularly, I maintained an excellent level of flexibility. When the hip doctor gave me his routine exam, he was surprised by how flexible I was. I told him that stretching helps with all of my discomforts. Since I had such a good range of motion, he completely dismissed me and my complaints about my hip pain. He told me that if I had a real hip issue, I wouldn't be able to have such good flexion. So, my pain was a figment of my imagination? I wanted to slap him. He's still a pretty popular guy in our community. All I think about when his name comes up is my desire to slap him.

After our daughter was born, I decided to go back to school to get a degree in cosmetology. At that time, Mark was buying the salon from his folks, so I wanted to be properly qualified to help him in any way possible. I was going to school full time, working as much as possible doing nails at the salon, still working out regularly, and, of course, raising the kids. It was a really hectic time in our lives, but we had an agenda. I could handle work and school, but it was important that our kids were taken care of. We hired a nanny full time that came to the house during the day. We were also extremely blessed because Mark's parents were unbelievably supportive and helpful with the kids. It also helped that they lived so close by.

Although I was overloaded, I didn't mind it. I have always thrived on being productive. Looking back, I imagine I was pushing myself pretty hard, but I had a goal in mind, and I was determined to reach that goal. Besides, if I kept busy, I didn't have to deal with any of the bad shit that happened. And, let's face it, we had a lot of bad shit happen.

By the third pregnancy a few years later, living in constant pain was getting the best of me. We decided that we wouldn't have any more than three children, because I couldn't handle all of the pain that accompanied my pregnancies. Once our third child Zachary was born, I was determined to figure out what the hell was wrong with me. Working full-time and being an active mother of three shouldn't have been this hard or this exhausting. I always had a good attitude, but the pain really sucked.

It was time to get an answer.

CHAPTER 6

SEARCHING FOR AN ANSWER

When I think about all the physical problems I've dealt with over the years, it is a wonder that I haven't gone a little bat-shit crazy. I have seen so many doctors in my lifetime, it'd make your head spin. I'd hate to tally all the co-pays I've spent, because it would probably make me cry. It feels like every time I sit down to work on this book, I remember another medicine, physician, or treatment. It's difficult to even remember all the doctors I've seen, but I remember enough to hopefully give you an idea of how difficult this journey for an answer has been for me.

More importantly, I hope I can guide you to find some answers of your own.

After our third child was born, I was working full-time at the salon with my husband as a nail technician. I was doing a lot of artificial nails and enjoyed growing my clientele.

Unfortunately, filing nails is repetitive and very strenuous on the arms, hands, and neck. It got to the point where my hands were going numb quite a bit of the time and I was constantly dropping things. My doctor sent me to a neurologist to get a nerve conduction test done. Basically, the doctor hooked me up to a machine that sent electrical currents through my hands. As soon as he turned on the machine, I started crying hysterically. Not only was the pain indescribable, but it was also emotionally upsetting because it felt like I was being electrocuted. After what happened to my father, I had a difficult time dealing with anything related to electricity. Can you blame me?

He was surprised by my reaction and told me that he had never seen anyone get that upset having the test done before. I'm not kidding when I tell you that nerve conduction tests hurt like a bitch. He told me I had moderate bilateral carpal tunnel syndrome. Surgery would have been a possibility only if I planned to change careers. If I continued at the salon, however, he told me I would probably just reinjure my hands again and would be back to square one.

Therefore, he recommended physical therapy.

The hand massages at physical therapy felt pretty good because they increased the circulation in my hands, but the exercises hurt a lot and actually did more harm than good. What I discovered was that the exercises caused a great deal of inflammation in my hands and wrists and actually exacerbated the pain and numbness. It was obvious that physical therapy was aggravating me more than anything. Even the therapist could tell that the exercises probably weren't helping, but they were determined to try to help me.

It's frustrating when a doctor tells you that physical therapy is the only answer while everything that was happening with my body was telling me that the therapy was doing more harm than good. I knew I should have listened to my body, but I was desperate for relief. I would later discover that my body gets inflamed very easily, and certain types of therapy, like physical therapy and chiropractic adjustments, make it worse. At the time, I would have done anything to get all of the feeling back in my hands, because it was becoming quite debilitating. So, I continued to go to PT even though I didn't think it was helping me because I was determined to get better so I could continue to service my nail clients. As you can probably imagine, it was a very frustrating time for me personally and professionally.

Carpal tunnel is really annoying. Sometimes, the simplest of activities were difficult. I remember trying to spoon spaghetti sauce into a bowl, and I dropped the ladle on the floor. Of course, it had to be red sauce that splattered all over the place. It was a huge mess, which made me cry. My husband told me to stop crying and just ask him to do things that are difficult. He is so sweet and supportive, but I'm an independent kind of gal and didn't expect my hands to not cooperate. Besides, I have a hard head and wanted to do it by myself. But man, red sauce can really splatter. It's the strangest sensation to have your hands go numb, and there was little I could do to make them feel better. It was really uncomfortable at night, which is how it all started. I tried a variety of braces, but they didn't help. My hands and often my forearms would still go numb even with the braces on and it was impossible to sleep because it was so uncomfortable.

As my condition worsened, I suffered with numbness and pain during the day as well.

One day, the therapist said he wanted to try something new, so he put my hands in gloves that looked like oven mitts. I assumed they would be hot. Boy was I wrong. As the mitts filled up, I felt the coldest sensation engulf my hands and forearms. At first, I was shocked by the way it felt, since I was expecting heat. Within moments, I realized I couldn't tolerate what was happening. It was the most pain I had ever felt in my hands, and I started to scream. It felt like someone was sawing my hands off. They pulled the mitts off immediately and wrapped my hands in warm towels to calm them (and me) down. It took me several minutes to stop crying.

The room was full of other patients, and everyone was staring at me. It was embarrassing, but I couldn't help myself. They said they never had anyone react that way to the mitts before, although some patients have complained in the past that the cold was uncomfortable. Uncomfortable is not what I felt. I felt brutally assaulted by a damn oven mitt. I always had a strange sensitivity to cold, but this treatment was completely unbearable and barbaric. That was the last time I went for physical therapy for my hands.

At the time, I was fortunate to have a client that owned a wellness center in our city who offered to help me. She knew I was struggling with the carpal tunnel, so she gave me a free acupuncture session. I had never had acupuncture before, but I was game to try anything. At the rate I was going, I was going to have to find a different career. After the first session, I had this strange sensation of my blood flowing through my hands and forearms. It was freaky and cool at the same time. I could literally feel blood flow to my semi-numb extremities. I wasn't sure about this acupuncture thing when I went into it, but I quickly became a believer.

A few hours after my first session, Mark and I drove to Buffalo to have dinner with my family. He drove most of the time back then because it was difficult for me to drive with numb hands. At one point during the drive, I told him that I wanted to tell him something, but I didn't want him to think I was crazy. He gave me that look. You know, the look like he already knew I was a bit crazy and loved me anyway… I told him that I felt like I was hallucinating because I could feel the blood flowing in my hands and forearms. He said he was happy for me, and whether or not he thought I was crazy, I'll never know. It didn't matter, because I did feel the blood flow into my hands. It was incredible.

After the second session, I had feelings in my hands again on a more regular basis, which made the pain lessen. I started reading more about this incredible treatment because it was more effective than anything else I had tried. Acupuncture was my new best friend. It was amazing!

Now that I found acupuncture as an alternative, I was finding some relief in my hands, and work became easier. I did not, however, know what the hell was wrong with the rest of my weird body. I had difficulty sleeping and was still having the night terrors. I felt like I had the flu a lot of the time, which I knew I didn't, but it was the way I felt. Every time I went to my primary physician, he wanted to give me some kind of medication hoping to placate me. In desperation, I tried several medications over the years, but they were all a bust.

One of the first medications I tried was amitriptyline. At the time, it was the most prescribed drug for people who suffered from fibromyalgia (even though I hadn't been diagnosed with it yet). When that proved to be more harmful than good, I was put on trazodone. They're both antidepressants that were supposed to help me sleep. Sadly, they made me groggy and didn't help me sleep. Instead, they made me depressed. Aside from my stint in Lynchburg, it was the only other time in my life I felt legitimately depressed. Within six weeks of trying each med, I was crying and sad a lot of the time. I couldn't even watch some commercials on the television without getting choked up. I got off of those meds before I became suicidal. I could not understand why anybody would want to take this shit.

I tried a plethora of pain medications because I was in pain so much of the time. Unfortunately, every pain medicine I tried ripped my stomach to shreds and did very little to relieve any of the pain. Substituting one pain for another never made any sense to me, so I usually gave up pretty quickly after trying each one. I remember my primary doctor suggesting a drug that he pretty much guaranteed wouldn't cause me abdominal distress and would make me more comfortable. It was called Meloxicam. Not only did it make me violently ill, it didn't touch the pain. At this point, you have to wonder why I tried so many things since everything always made me so sick. I'll tell you why. I hurt—real, honest-to-goodness pain—and I was looking for some kind of relief. There were so many times over the years that I felt an urgent sense of desperation and was willing to try practically anything.

Over-the-counter and prescription painkillers were both recommended, such as Tylenol, Advil, Naproxen, and Aleve… Yep, I have popped a lot of pills in my lifetime. Sadly, they didn't get rid of the pain, and almost every single one of them caused secondary issues. That didn't make sense to me. So, my back might hurt less but now my stomach was wrecked? It wasn't worth the tradeoff. To this day, I have to laugh when I listen to all of the side effects that medications can cause. I'll stick with the primary issue, since some of the side effects are so extreme—like death. Yeah, I'll pass on that.

I tried muscle relaxers to help with all of the muscle pain, however I didn't like feeling like I had no control. Besides, they never made the pain any less. I do think that the dosage was too high because I can tolerate muscle relaxers now. The crazy thing was that back then, the muscle relaxers actually made me anxious. When you're a productive woman who likes to be in control, medications designed to help you relax can have the opposite effect. I didn't like my limbs feeling even weaker than they normally were. And they didn't help me sleep, so what was the point? They also made me feel goofy in the head, which freaked me out. The doctor told me my muscles wouldn't heal if they didn't have the chance to relax. Heal from what? Yes, that reasoning was very plausible, but it wasn't as easily achieved as one would think. Besides, I still didn't have any kind of rational explanation as to why they hurt in the first place.

Since I still experienced some nerve pain in my hands and often my neck, my doctor prescribed Neurontin, which is commonly used for nerve pain. I read up on the drug and discovered it was a medication that was developed for the brain, but, once again, I was desperate for some relief. At this point in my life, my head was still the only thing that didn't hurt. By day three, I couldn't put on mascara because there were psychedelic waves in front of my face. It felt like I was on some kind of LSD trip. When I went to work, I tried to wax a woman's eyebrows and it was impossible because of all the floaters impairing my vision. It didn't take long for me to realize that Neurontin was not the drug for me. It was scary as hell, and I threw the bottle away.

At one point, I went through my medicine cabinet and was floored by the dozens of bottles of prescriptions that I had tried and didn't continue to take because the side effects were so difficult on my system. Since I never took any one drug for very long, I had forgotten about many of them. To this day, I'm still baffled by how many different prescriptions I tried. It made me feel very uneasy. Was I really this fucked up? This whole situation regarding my body and my health was frustrating beyond belief. I wasted a lot of money on useless drugs, which made me a huge skeptic about any prescription medicine. It was a discouraging revelation to know that something was wrong and that the two dozen bottles of pills in my cabinet were not even remotely the answer.

When I complained to my doctor again, he decided that my nutrition must be lacking and that was why I didn't feel good. He gave me the name of a nutritionist. When I called to make an appointment with her, she told me to log everything that went into my mouth for two weeks and she would review it when we met and figure out what was lacking in my diet or what changes needed to be made. She emphasized that I even needed to write down if I chewed gum or had a breath mint. Ironically, I don't like sucking on hard candy or mints, and gum bothers my teeth and jaw, so there was no need to jot any of those kinds of things down. I wasn't kidding; I am ridiculously sensitive to pretty much every place on my body.

It was a pain to write everything down, but I was hoping she could figure something out for me. During this time in my life, I was reading a lot about holistic medicine, Chinese medicine, and even nutrition. I have a huge collection of self-help and informational books. I definitely was skeptical about being nutritionally deficient, but I was secretly hoping she'd find something obvious in my diet that was causing all my issues. One could only hope, right?

When I handed her my journal two weeks later, she spent about ten minutes reviewing everything I ate. It felt weird watching her dissect my diet, and I worried that she might judge me. I didn't know anything about her, and I wasn't sure what kind of nutritional path in life she followed because there are so many different schools of thought regarding the best diets you should follow. After she got to the end of my list, she looked up at me and said, "Why are you here?" I told her that I lived in constant pain and always felt like I had the flu, and since my doctor couldn't figure out what was wrong with me, he suggested I see a nutritionist to detect whether or not some kind of nutritional deficiency might be the problem. She told me that she doubted my diet was the problem. In fact, she said, "You have a better diet than I do." I remember her saying that like it was yesterday.

At this point in my life, I was very conscientious about what I ate, so I had to laugh when she told me I had a better diet than she did. I wasn't surprised. Aside from my fast-food junky days in college, I was a healthy eater. Well, it was time to scratch that explanation off my list.

She had no recommendations for me and didn't want to accept me as a patient. So, now what?

Since I complained about the pains in my joints, my doctor thought it might be a good idea to see a rheumatologist. Whoopee, another freaking doctor! Blood work didn't show any arthritis at this time in my life but there was a new condition called fibromyalgia that the doctor thought might be the cause of my problems. I wasn't exactly sure what fibromyalgia was, but, at that time, rheumatologists were the only doctors who could accurately diagnose the condition. When I looked up fibro on the Internet, it sounded very obscure, and there was little information about it. From the description I read, I wasn't very clear about what it was, but it sounded like the kind of thing that could possibly describe what I had been experiencing for most of my life. Since there was so little online about this newly diagnosed ailment, I had no idea how they tested for it or what it really meant.

When I met with the rheumatologist, she asked me why I was there. I told her, "My doctor can't figure out what is wrong with me, and at this point, I'm convinced he thinks I'm crazy." Although I was discouraged, I always maintained a sense of humor and tried to keep some levity in the discussions regarding my issues. To this day, that has remained my approach because it is the coping mechanism that seems to work best for me. Meeting another doctor and whining about my situation wasn't who I was, and it still isn't who I am. I gave her the rundown of all my maladies and the various doctors I had met with over the years. I even tried to regurgitate the names of the countless medications I tried. Every time I went through this discussion, I started to doubt the validity of my ailments more and more. Maybe my issues were a bit psychosomatic, since no one could pinpoint the crux of my pain or discomfort. She asked me if they suspected I had fibromyalgia. I told her that I had no idea, but maybe that was why he sent me to her. All I did know was that my primary physician kept sending me to different healthcare practitioners because my complaints didn't make sense, and he didn't have any answers. I guess you could say he was passing the buck, and I was so frustrated that I wanted to tell everyone to "buck off."

To put things into perspective, it was the year 2000. I had just finished dealing with a debilitating bout of anxiety that put me in the hospital. Between all the catastrophic rumors surrounding the new millennium and all the shit I was dealing with in my life, I was legitimately falling apart. Experiencing extreme anxiety coupled with chronic panic attacks is crippling. I thought I was dying. My mom had to live with us and help me with our children for a short time because I was having panic attacks on a regular basis—like every fifteen minutes. All of the shit in my life came to a head, and I was falling apart. I needed answers now more than ever. Maybe this woman could shed some light on my situation.

It felt strange seeing a rheumatologist since I didn't have arthritis (at least I didn't think I did). She told me that I looked great (although it was flattering, I was sick of hearing that) and that she found it very unlikely I had fibro because I didn't fit the "profile" of a typical fibro patient. Apparently, since I wasn't overweight, lethargic, or depressed, it was doubtful that I had this condition. Although I was in constant pain, none of those adjectives were characteristics of my personality. I was always a high-energy, positive person who refused to succumb to my maladies despite how crappy I felt—except for my short bout with anxiety. Fortunately, it was a brief stint, and I was able to get through it pretty quickly. At this point in my professional life, I worked at the salon full time, and I prided myself on looking my best at all times—in and out of work. Besides, the better I looked, the better I felt. Even though the bout of anxiety set me back a few weeks for the first time in my life, I fought to get right back on track, and I did. I wasn't letting panic attacks, or any other ailment, take me down. If it wasn't a life-threatening disease, I was determined to win—no matter what it took.

Testing for fibro is random and obscure, and I still can't believe they haven't come up with a more accurate diagnostic technique. It's also subjective. I believe that if her approach to the test had been gentler or more aggressive, then the result and further diagnosis could have been different. The doctor told me she would be touching different spots on my body to see if I had sensitivity to any of them. She referred to this exam as a tender point test. There were eighteen spots that ranged from my feet to my neck. If eleven were tender, then my fibro test would be positive. It was hard not to laugh at the absurdity of this kind of testing and I still shake my head over it. Getting poked on my skin with one of her fingers didn't sound very legitimate or diagnostic, and it seemed comical that this trained professional was actually going to do this to me.

First, she touched a spot on my ankle, and I couldn't believe how much it hurt. When she touched the second spot on the inside of my knee, my leg shot forward and I yelped in pain and started to cry, mostly because I kicked her and was embarrassed by my reaction. I couldn't help it. It hurt and I couldn't control my response. She touched the most bizarre spots on my body and every single one was extremely painful. Although I was skeptical of this bizarre tender point test, I definitely reacted to each and every point that she touched. Every spot she put pressure on was sensitive to the touch. I couldn't believe how bizarre this whole thing was, and it was disconcerting that such random places on my body were so sensitive to her touch. I knew I had weird sensitivities, but this was freaky.

When she finished her exam, she sat down, crossed her legs, and shook her head in disbelief. She told me that she expected the exam to produce negative results because of how I looked, how productive I was, and how much energy

I had. As it turned out, all eighteen tender points on my body were positively responsive to her touch. She couldn't believe it. She said she never met anyone who was eighteen for eighteen. Gee, I always need to be special, don't I? She reiterated the point that she never expected me to have the condition, but the test could not have been more conclusive. Although I looked good, my body was a hot mess. Finally, an answer (or so I thought…).

After she made her diagnosis, she wrote down some notes and sat there quietly for a minute. I waited for her to say something. Finally, she reiterated that I did indeed have this strange condition called fibromyalgia, and she was sorry to tell me that there was nothing she could do for me. Wait…what did she just say? WTF! She continued by saying there was no course of treatment at this time for fibro and no specific doctor who could deal with my issues. This was in 2000. Medications could be prescribed, but they would probably just mask my symptoms and potentially cause me more problems. She offered to write me any kind of prescription I felt I needed, but there were none I wanted to try. I had never found any medication in the past that gave me relief, so I had no desire to try anymore.

At one point during our consultation, she asked me if I was a vegetarian. Ironically, at the time, I was and had been since I was pregnant with my second child. She recommended that I start adding animal protein to my diet again because it tended to build stronger muscles, and I needed to protect my fragile joints. I told her that I had a hard time digesting meat and there were certain meats that I would never consume again. She suggested I do small amounts, like three to four ounces at a time, and see how I feel. I reintroduced meat into my diet again after I met with her, but it didn't seem to make a difference one way or the other about the way I felt.

She also recommended I take glucosamine-chondroitin daily. I needed to take 1,500 mg of the one and 1,250 of the other for it to be effective. I agreed because she said it could help my knee, which was always a source of pain. I took that supplement for over ten years until I developed arthritis, and it got so bad that the supplement had no effect on me anymore. In the beginning, it did have an analgesic effect, so I made sure I took three pills every morning. After time wore on, however, it stopped helping.

She also reiterated how important it was for me to get daily exercise. She was preaching to the choir there because exercise was my saving grace and an important part of my daily regimen. She did tell me she was impressed with my dedication to exercise since most people in chronic pain couldn't deal with adding exercise to their life and usually lacked the motivation or energy to start any workout program. I told her that increasing my circulation helped with the pain and numbness, and frankly, I don't deal well with being overweight. Extra weight puts more stress on your joints which worsens the pain so trying to stay fit needs to be a priority.

Not only did she tell me there was nothing she could do for me, but she also said that unless I had an arthritic concern, she couldn't see me as a patient anymore. That was difficult to hear. At this point, there were few treatments for people with fibromyalgia because it was such a new and unknown condition, so it didn't make any sense for her to see me anyway. I understood her rationale, but I didn't like it. I seemed to have mastered walking into brick walls. No wonder I have such a small nose.

At the time, many doctors were prescribing amitriptyline to help with the sleep disorders that accompany fibro, but I had already tried it and it was a disaster. As I stated earlier, I tried a six-week course of two different antidepressants, and they both made me depressed. Furthermore, they didn't help me sleep so it made no sense to stay on either of them. The rheumatologist told me she had ten thousand arthritis patients and didn't have room for any fibro patients. In addition, she told me there would be difficulties with my insurance covering my doctor visits since no one was quite sure what category it fell under. I thanked her and left her office feeling empty and confused.

I finally had an answer, but I didn't have anyone who could help me manage it. I had fibromyalgia. Of course, I had a whack-a-doodle condition with some weird name attached to it that no one had a clue how to deal with. I'd never been normal up to this point, so why would I have a normal disease? It was the new millennium, and I had this problem that nobody could help me with. It didn't make sense. I was happy to have a name to it but equally as frustrated to be forced to deal with it on my own. I had been living with inexplicable pain since 1978 and I finally had an answer. There was a part of me that was relieved and another part that was annoyed as hell. I knew I had to deal with this head-on and figure out how to deal with this newfound knowledge. The problem was, what the fuck was fibro?

The research that I found online was intermittent and confusing. I read about widespread pain, nerve disorders, weakness, difficulties sleeping, flu-like symptoms, and problems concentrating. Yep, that sounded about right. The cause was unknown. The treatment was unknown. It figures I'd have something nutty like this. It made sense though. I did have everything that they described except the personality and attitude that often accompanied people like me. From my online research, fibro patients were almost always referred to as depressed, not physically fit, and lethargic, just like the rheumatologist had said to me, which is why no one would have suspected I had it. Screw that. I never wanted any of those characteristics to be attributed to me. It was a frustrating consultation, to say the least, but I was impressed with how much time she spent with me. I was in the exam room for close to an hour, which is unheard of these days. You're lucky if you get ten minutes with a doctor. This lady was amazing and I'm sorry she has since retired. I have to admit that I wasn't happy about her explanation of my situation, but I was relieved to know I wasn't crazy. I decided that it was time to be even more proactive and figure out how I was going to overcome this ridiculous-sounding thing I had. Fibro the fuck myalgia!

CHAPTER 7

NOW WHAT?

After twenty-two years, I had a name associated with all of the problems I had been dealing with since middle school. So what? It really didn't change anything. That was psychologically and emotionally difficult to process. I always assumed if a physician could figure out the cause of my maladies, there would be an answer. Well, guess who was the ass with that assumption? The only good thing about the diagnosis was that it reiterated the fact that I was not a hypochondriac and still am not. Believe me, there have been countless times over the years when I thought that maybe I was being oversensitive to the strange sensations I experienced. Sometimes I even questioned if my pain was a little bit fabricated, and I used it as a coping strategy to deal with stress or even get out of stressful situations. I never was the kind of person to doubt myself, but after so many years of chronic pain, doubting the validity of my problems was becoming a real thing. There was some comfort in acknowledging to myself that I wasn't being a crybaby, and I really did have something wrong with me. Even if it was difficult to pronounce and even more difficult to spell. It was a relief to know I wasn't crazy despite there being no doctors that would be willing to take me on as a patient. And let's not forget that there was no treatment. It was a very conflicting time in my life.

Since I had tried different approaches to dealing with my issues in the past, I couldn't see anything different for the future, which was frustrating. In fact, I feared that things would continue to get more difficult as I got older and that was really scary. There was no way this was going to get any better in the future unless I found some way to make the symptoms less pronounced. Although it was disheartening, I was never a quitter, and I had to remain diligent about being in control of my well-being (or lack thereof).

One day I got a call from my mother. She told me that a local doctor from her community decided to switch from Western Medicine to alternative medicine. He was a general surgeon in her community who completely gave up his practice because he was discouraged with the way the future of our medical community was heading. He had actually done surgery on my grandfather's hip a few years before that, and I remember meeting him in the hospital. My mother informed me that he was doing treatments for people with various ailments, including fibro. I decided to give him a try.

This guy impressed me from the moment I met him. He said that he was tired of treating the symptoms that his patients came to him with and was more interested in finding the cause of their problems. For example, if someone had chronic sinus or bronchial infections, he wanted to figure out what was causing the infections. Was it dust, mold, or some type of allergen causing the infections? Or was an abundance of yeast causing the excess inflammation that was triggering the infections? I liked that he was trying to find the root of people's problems instead of just prescribing a pill to mask the symptoms or temporarily fix the ailment. This especially pleased me since I never had any luck with pills. To this day, I have never met a general practitioner that has been so interested in "why" I got sick. I find most doctors still like to prescribe medication.

After a thorough consultation about everything that was going on in my body, he believed that injections of hydrogen peroxide were the most effective way of cleaning out my system and helping to minimize the pain and flu-like symptoms I was experiencing. I would sit for two hours at a time and have hydrogen peroxide injected into my system. I can't say I felt any better with the treatments, but I was willing to try it for several months. I also had infusions of pure oxygen, which gave me bursts of sunshine and energy. He would take a blood sample, infuse it with O3, and inject it back into my system. Now *that* felt amazing. I also received injections of glutathione, which made me feel great as well. I wasn't cured, but I felt a little better after the treatments.

I have to thank my mother for all of her support during these sessions. They were very expensive, and she helped me pay for them. She would also meet me at the facility, since it was closer to her house than mine, and it would give us the chance to spend time together. I can't remember how many hours I sat in that room, but it was a lot. I was grateful that my husband supported me during all of these crazy treatments. It has to be extremely hard for anyone to really understand what another person is going through, especially when the pain isn't visual. He'd drive an hour and a half with me one way on our day off so that I could sit in a chair and get strange solutions pumped through my body. Now is that love or what?

At one point during my time with this doctor, he suggested I have a bio-feedback test. It was a diagnostic tool that was becoming popular on the West Coast of the US but hadn't hit the East Coast yet. Apparently, there were situations where people would get very ill, and no one could figure out the cause of the ailment. This machine could help discover the crux of the problem. It sounded bizarre, but I had nothing to lose. He explained that the technician would hook me up to a computer and get diagnostic findings that may help us discern where all the pain was originating. There was no pain involved with the testing, and the test didn't take very long.

What did I have to lose?

The only thing the technician knew about me was that my name was Mary. He didn't know anything else about me and he had no idea what ailments I was suffering from. He hooked my fingers up to electrodes that were connected to his computer. A few minutes into the test, he made a comment that surprised me. He said, "You must get the flu vaccine." It was a flat statement with zero emotion attached to it.

"Why?" I asked him. He continued to press buttons, and the whole thing seemed a little strange.

"You have an extremely high level of the flu virus in your system," he replied—again with no emotional effect attached to the statement

"That must explain why I feel like I have the flu so much of the time?" I asked him. At first, he didn't say anything. I had continued to get the flu shot through my third pregnancy because my doctor recommended it. It never occurred to me not to get it. I asked the technician if I should stop getting the flu shot; he told me that he was simply a technician and wasn't qualified to make a diagnosis or any recommendations. He was just letting me know what the test was showing. It seemed pretty obvious to me that the flu shot was poisoning me.

Between the traumas from my father's accident, the incident with my dog, and the flu vaccine every year since my first child was born, I *had* been feeling flu-ish on a regular basis.

That was probably my biggest complaint. I never put the combination of the above factors as a cause for my pain. Things were getting more interesting. I started feeling like I had some control over my body. If the flu shot was poisoning me, then that was something I could eliminate from my yearly doctor visit.

From that point on, I stopped getting the flu shot. It wasn't as easy as I thought it would be to stop getting it, however. My regular doctor kept insisting that I get the shot. He believed that anyone with fibro who worked with the public must be vaccinated yearly. I understood that I had a weakened immune system and couldn't risk getting the flu, but I truly believed the shot was not helping me and was, in fact, making me more unwell. He told me that it could be very dangerous if I got the flu, and that I could even end up in the hospital. When I explained the testing I had done at the clinic in Buffalo, he didn't believe it was an accurate form of diagnosis and thought the whole biofeedback testing system was bunk. He was fairly adamant about me getting vaccinated. Even though I was uncomfortable, I stood up for myself and told him that I wouldn't let him give it to me.

In order to get him to stop bugging me about it, I did something extremely uncharacteristic; I told him my gynecologist gave me the flu shot. That wasn't true. I have told very few lies in my lifetime, but I felt like I had no choice. In most circumstances, I tell the truth regardless of the outcome. I'd rather suffer the wrath of being completely honest, no matter what. But in this instance, I found it easier to tell him I got the shot so he wouldn't criticize me. I just didn't have the energy to keep defending my opinion. Ultimately, it's my body and I should do what I think is right for me, don't you think? He believed the test was a lot of nonsense and felt that my reasoning was unsubstantiated. It made me feel uncomfortable telling him the lie year after year, but he didn't believe in the biofeedback testing that I did. In his mind, the explanation wasn't plausible, and he was steadfast in his conviction that I should get the flu vaccine every year.

I've gotten much stronger about standing up for myself since then. Now, I just say no to the flu shot. I don't want it and I shouldn't have to explain my reasoning. That's the beauty of getting older and not allowing another person to make decisions that affect my health. I definitely think the flu shot made my symptoms worse and I refuse to inject that poison into my system anymore. It is my body and my decision. End of story.

But I'm still achy. Not all of the time, but randomly. When I feel like the flu is consuming my limbs, I suffer. Anyone would. It's real and it's exhausting. Sometimes the ache can be so debilitating that it makes it difficult to function. Other times, it's just annoying, like a toothache. Instead of succumbing to the feeling, however, it has been my quest for years to figure out what triggers my flare-ups and the best way to combat the discomfort. There is something very powerful about listening to your body and paying attention to what it is trying to tell you.

Let's be honest, most of us are not good listeners when it comes to our bodies.

For the record, that is what we fibro sufferers call it when we have a painful episode—a flare-up. Our body experiences some kind of change that triggers a physical response of pain, numbness, or lethargy. Flare-ups can range from being annoying to absolutely debilitating. They affect your skin, sleep, cognition, mood, sensitivity to smells, light, and sound. This is an all-encompassing condition that can really knock you on your ass. The most important component in my mind is to determine the catalyst that triggered the flare-up and decide the best way to deal with it. Do you crawl under the covers and hide, or do you face it head-on and say *f' you, fibro?* I think it's pretty obvious how I approach it (most of the time, that is).

One thing I'd like you to remember is that some of the remedies that help me may not help you, and vice versa. I'm just sharing my story so you may find some relief and find more joy in your life. For example, some fibro sufferers are huge proponents of herbal therapy. That is awesome for them. For the most part, they don't help me. I've tried a variety of Chinese herbs that have wreaked total chaos in my body. For some reason, my system has difficulty assimilating many herbs, and I end up having some kind of negative response. So, you need to know that my goal is to offer suggestions, motivation, and empathy, because I get it. I really do. You are not alone; I know your pain is real, and I care, which is why I've dedicated myself to writing this memoir.

My primary goal and focus for as long as I can remember has been to keep a positive attitude despite my continuous aches and pains. This single component (my positive attitude) has probably been my savior throughout this whole journey. In spite of how shitty I feel, I was raised to focus on the positive and I have tried to do that no matter how bleak things seem or how shitty I feel. Don't get me wrong, I moan and groan now and again, but then I kick myself in my ass and focus on thinking about the good things in my life and not dwell on my shortcomings. Someone always has it worse than me, and fibro is not life-threatening. These are two very important things that you need to tell yourself each and every day.

In spite of how difficult living with fibro has been at times, I have tried to be diligent about having control of my body to the best of my ability. I have never fully succumbed to my predicament, because I've been persistent in my pursuit of living a pain-free and happy life. It has been a constant battle because I don't want to always feel this way. One of the problems, however, is that I keep getting injured, and that has screwed up my plans to overcome this weird condition I have. Since our fundamental structures are more fragile, we tend to get hurt more often—at least that is my experience. I can list a problem with more parts of my body than you can imagine. It's my normal, and it may be yours as well. But these are the cards we have been dealt and I think it is vital that we deal with our condition head-on and not let it take over our lives in such a drastic way that we are unable to find any joy in our life.

You've probably noticed by now that I don't refer to fibromyalgia as a disease. In my mind, diseases are often life-threatening, and although fibro can be debilitating, it rarely is fatal (which is something I will reiterate until I am blue in the face and will remind you of repeatedly throughout this book). Complications from fibro and the medications used to treat the symptoms can escalate and cause secondary issues that can be life-threatening, and sadly that is one of the risks we may have to face if we take a lot of prescription medications. Unfortunately, there are a lot of medications that are being prescribed that can be more dangerous than good—like when I took Neuroton that caused dizziness and impaired my eyesight. It doesn't mean that many of you wouldn't be able to function with medication, but if you're taking something that may or may not help and isn't necessary for your survival, I'd love for you to rethink the efficacy of what you are taking.

There are so many meds that I tried that were supposed to mask some of my symptoms, but they ended up causing more debilitating secondary problems that I've become a huge skeptic. For example, I have osteoarthritis. If there isn't a drug on the market that will slow down the progression, then what's the point? I'm better off doing more yoga and swimming even more because "motion is lotion," especially when you grow older and are arthritic.

If you haven't figured it out by now, it's your mindset that I'm appealing to. You have the power to be happy or the power to be miserable. It's all up to you. You and you alone. That is one of the main reasons I chose to write this book. I want to alter the mindset of those who suffer from this affliction and help people feel better so they can enjoy more fulfilling lives.

But the injuries keep interrupting my campaign to feel better, which made my path to wellness more complicated. For example, in 2008, I herniated a disc in my neck. I had been having neck and shoulder pain for some time and wasn't surprised when the injury happened. I was waxing a woman and suddenly felt an excruciating stab in the back of my neck. The pain was so intense that it brought tears to my eyes. Even though I was only halfway through her service, I was determined to finish. I had to take a minute to compose myself when the injury happened because the pain was so intense, so I turned away from her, feigning the excuse that I needed to change my gloves. It was the only stalling technique I could come up with while my eyes dried and I could catch my breath.

When I finally finished the client, I took four Advil and finished my day in utter misery. At one point, Mark found me in the kitchen with my head down on the table. When he asked what was wrong, I told him I was sore from waxing one of my clients. At the time, I suspected it was muscular. Boy was I wrong. I drank a lot of wine that night and went to bed early because it hurt to hold my head up. The next morning, I couldn't lift my head off of my pillow. I was really scared. Mark had to physically get me to the standing position. This was definitely more serious than a pissed-off muscle, and I knew I needed to see someone. I went to the hospital and had an MRI; it showed I had herniated the disc between my C5 and C6 vertebrae. I couldn't believe it.

This injury was real.

When the doctor asked me how I hurt myself I told him I did it by "waxing a forty-seven-year-old Italian lady's vagina." I think I sounded like a whiny version of Lucille Ball when I said that to him because I emphasized the word vagina in a very high-pitched and whiny tone. Suddenly he was worried that this was a workman's compensation case and asked me if it was since it happened at work. I assured him it was our salon, not a workman's comp case, and to focus on my neck and not to worry about the insurance. I have to say it was pretty obvious he wasn't sure how to react to my frankness about how the herniation happened. He was obviously young and new to medicine, and it was comical to see how he tried to remain professional as he processed how the injury occurred. Aside from the pain and the fear associated with the diagnosis, one of my basic coping skills has been to maintain a sense of humor, and I did, in fact, hurt myself by giving a forty-seven-year-old Italian woman a Brazilian bikini wax. Since my honesty made him visibly uncomfortable, he basically ignored it and told me my options. He explained that there was a herniation between two of the discs in my neck, which was very serious. He believed that surgery was the best answer.

Fortunately, my husband cut the hair of a prominent orthopedic surgeon in town at the time. Even though it was a Sunday, he called this doctor and told him what happened. He firmly told Mark to make sure this man did NOT perform any type of surgery on me. The doctor on call was young and inexperienced, and that was the last person I wanted to cut me—especially in the neck. We appreciated his honesty and scheduled an appointment with the orthopedic surgeon the following day.

He recommended me to one of his colleagues that specialized in the neck and back. At first, the injury was causing me serious impairment and excruciating pain and it was difficult to function, so I felt compelled to have it fixed. The surgeon showed me the pictures from the MRI, explained what the problem was in detail, and gave me all of my options. He told me that countless people function with herniated discs, and I may feel better once the inflammation goes down. When it first happened, however, I couldn't handle how much it hurt. On the other hand, neck surgery is scary, and I knew I had to be tough and ride it out until the inflammation and pain lessened.

I decided to forego surgery and live with the pain since surgery was risky and would be a temporary fix. After a few years, it continued to hurt most of the time, and I just wanted the pain to stop. I went back to the surgeon and told him I couldn't take it anymore. He explained how he would make an incision in the front of my neck, which could impair my voice or in the worst-case scenario, cut my vocal cords and hinder my ability to ever speak again. Some surgeons prefer to make the incision in the back of the neck, but that technique can cause paralysis. Let's see, would I prefer to not be able to speak or to not be able to walk? Both options sucked, but I favored the speaking one. Then he would put a cadaver bone between the discs to give the area more stability. When I went for the pre-operative appointment, they told me I had to have a nerve conduction test on my spine prior to the surgery. As I previously mentioned I had a similar test on my hands, and I was irrational when it happened. I couldn't handle the pain. The physician's assistant also remarked that we needed to hope that the surgery would last for ten years. I was dumbfounded. I thought it was a one-time thing. Wrong again. He explained that when you stabilize one area, the surrounding discs tend to weaken. This would be the first of many neck surgeries. Oh yeah, and there is always the risk of paralysis or permanent vocal damage. No thanks! I decided to live with it.

Instead of getting cut open and missing three weeks of work, I canceled the surgery, and we bought a hot tub instead. Heat does make it feel better (except when it causes more inflammation), but nothing is perfect. To this day, I go in our hot tub on a regular basis. Massage and heat may be Band-Aids, but they are Band-Aids that work well enough to keep me going.

Sadly, I had more crazy shit happen to my body after this incident that did require surgery.

One morning I was standing at my kitchen counter prepping food for a summer party we were having. We were expecting about thirty people at our house. At one point, I turned towards my fridge and couldn't bend my knee. I looked down and it was huge! You couldn't see any bones. It was just big and puffy. I yelled for Mark. "Now what did you do?" he asked. This poor man has had to deal with more problems with me. It's never-ending. Thank God he loves me!

"I didn't do anything!" I said, frustrated. I iced it a lot that day, but the swelling wouldn't go down. I had felt a clicking feeling in my knee for months, but it never occurred to me to get it checked out because my knees had been giving me trouble since I was thirteen years old. Fortunately, I was able to get into the orthopedic office the next day and see one of the PAs.

The X-ray showed nothing, so the doctor said I needed an MRI. I asked him what he thought it was and he said he suspected a tumor. I had the MRI a few days later and was scheduled to meet the surgeon the following Monday. It was the same surgeon we called when I herniated the disc in my neck. Sadly, the PA was right. Apparently, the synovial fluid in my knee developed a tumor that needed to be taken out or else I could potentially lose my leg. Oh, isn't that a happy thought? Believe me when I say that fear and stress are not friends to the fibro sufferer. When the surgeon cut me open, he discovered I had two forms of the disease in my knee, diffused and nodular. Not only had I never heard of the disease, I had two forms of it.

Couldn't I just have a normal meniscus tear like the average Joe?

They wanted me to take two weeks off of work, but that can be difficult when you're self-employed, so I only took one. As I was waxing one of my regular clients, I lost my balance and fell against the waxing table. The client (who

I knew was a physician) asked what happened. I told her I had knee surgery. "For what?" she asked.

"A condition called PVNS," I told her.

"Was it diffused or nodular?" she wanted to know.

"Both," I replied, surprised that she had heard of it.

"Did Dr. Bronstein do it?" she asked.

How would you know that? I wondered.

Apparently, she was the orthopedic oncologist called to consult on the case. Oncologist? What the heck! As it turns out, she specialized in the disease and has written several articles on the subject in medical journals. She told me that in the first two years, I had an 80 percent chance of the disease coming back, and after that I had a 45 percent chance of it recurring. And if it did come back then I would have major surgery where they would have to cut 50 percent of my leg open in both the front and the back, and then the entire area would need to be thoroughly irrigated. She said that if the surgery wasn't that thorough, the disease would basically eat my bones, and I'd lose my leg. The recovery was a minimum of six months, and I would be unable to work that entire time. No thanks, I'll pass. The only way to make sure the disease hasn't come back is by getting MRIs. She informed me that I needed to get continual MRIs every six months for a few years to ensure my knee was disease-free. I'm several years out since the surgery and things seem to be okay. Although the tumor was not cancer, it acts like cancer and can eat away at my bones. Yep, I'm the special one who gets a disease in my synovial fluid. WTF!

When the orthopedic surgeon fixed my knee, he said I had a lot of arthritis in there as well. It didn't surprise me since I had struggled with knee pain since I was a teenager. Now that I had a legitimate arthritic concern and a variety of other cranky parts, I decided to go back to the rheumatologist to get her assessment of the type of arthritis I had and whether or not it explained some of the other pain I had been dealing with. It was 2010—ten years after she diagnosed me with fibro.

When I walked into her office, she didn't seem surprised to see me. She confirmed that I had developed osteoarthritis in several parts of my body. I didn't get as upset as I thought I would, however. It wasn't rheumatoid arthritis, which can be crippling and, in the end, would be far more debilitating. It was osteoarthritis, and I needed to accept it as part of the aging process. Again, it could be worse. On the other hand, when she told me that my bone density had decreased, I lost it. I work out, lift weights, keep my weight down, eat a healthy diet, and my bones are *still* aging. God, that pissed me off. It was another reminder that I was losing control over my body, and I didn't like it at all.

Since then, I've developed arthritis in a few more parts of my body and have accepted it as part of the aging process. I'm still pissed off about the bone density, though. Bone loss equates to being old in my head. Fortunately, my last bone density test showed I was still in the normal range for a woman my age. Another small victory.

We talked about arthritis and then she asked me what I wanted to do about it. I told her I noticed that there were several medications advertised on television for osteoarthritis, and my question was whether or not any of the medications slowed down the progression of the disease or could help repair the bones from arthritis. She emphatically said no. The medications were all developed to mask the symptoms and did nothing to fix the problem, and, like most medications, there was always the risk of side effects. I told her I was not interested in taking any of them.

She asked me what my biggest complaint was. I didn't even have to think about that one. It's funny because one of the most annoying things that bugged me about developing arthritis was how symphonic my body sounded when I got up in the morning. Everything cracks from my neck, my back, my hips, my knees, and even my feet. The sound makes me feel old, and even if it doesn't really hurt, it sounds yucky. I think it is more psychologically painful than anything else. I can't stand how noisy I am. When your parts Snap, Crackle, and Pop (remember the Rice Krispies Cereal ad?), it is called crepitus. That's where the word decrepit comes from (a random fact I like sharing with others). It's a word I've used a lot since then because I really like saying it even though I don't like having it. Strange things amuse me… Anyways, the rheumatologist recommended that I take a supplement called hyaluronic acid. She told me that she had a noisy, arthritic body part that stopped making so much noise once she took this on a regular basis and was suggesting her patients try it. My concern was the side effects. If there were side effects to be had, I was the queen of all of them. Fortunately, a quieter body was the only side effect I had to worry about.

As it turns out, there is definitely something to this hyaluronic acid stuff. I'm ten years older since then, and my body still doesn't make as much noise. There is still some creaking, especially in my neck, but it is nothing like it used to be. Now I have to rely on good old-fashioned musical instruments if I want to hear a symphony.

She also suggested I start taking collagen powder. Once again, I asked her about the side effects. She said that the only thing she noticed was that many people commented that their hair gets thicker. For once, that was a side effect I could live with. Our skin and joints lose collagen as we age, so it was a really good idea to add it to my diet.

It's funny because they say that getting arthritis and experiencing declining bone density is all a part of the maturation process. For the record, I think being mature is highly overrated. I hate hearing people complain that getting old sucks, because what's the alternative? For the record, I would rather get older and try to find joy at every age then what…die? I hope to stick around as long as possible even with all my cranky parts.

I decided that it was time to do more research and see what other changes I could make in my life to slow down this aging body of mine as I was getting more pissed off by the minute. I don't like feeling old because I have an extremely youthful mind and attitude.

About a year later (I've never kept a journal so I'm approximating the time frame), I started having excruciating pain in my hands, particularly my fingers. I couldn't hold a coffee cup, wrap my hands around my steering wheel, or stick shift, and I can't even explain how difficult work was becoming. Finger pain would wake me up in the middle of the night. It wasn't numbness like when I had carpal tunnel; this was a whole new animal. I called the nurse at the rheumatology office and told her that I thought I had bone cancer in my hands and was freaking out. Okay, I admit I get a little irrational sometimes. With all the problems I've had, I surmise that you would get a little crazy now and again also. Anyway, she told me to come in at seven in the morning the following day and the doctor would look at me (by the way, this kind of attention made me love this doctor even more!). She took my hands in hers and said, "I don't think this is bone cancer. In fact, I'm confident that what you are dealing with now is a condition called De Quervain's tenosynovitis." Are you kidding me? What the hell was that? Apparently, the tendonitis in my wrists was so bad that it was causing transference pain and stiffness in my fingers. She ordered a boatful of blood work to rule out anything creepy just to placate me. She must have realized I needed reassurance. Besides, it's better to be safe…

She also recommended an anti-inflammatory medication, which I reluctantly agreed to take. It was the first time she suggested meds, so I decided to give it a go. Although my inflammation was visible, I was nervous about the side effects. Within a few days, this medication triggered explosive headaches whenever I exerted myself. Whenever I would climax, for example, I would get a crippling pain in my head. It was terrifying. Furthermore, all the blood vessels in my eye broke while I was sleeping, and I didn't have a clue what was happening to me. I went to an eye doctor who said he suspected that I had a brain aneurysm. Now I was completely freaked out. Fortunately, my husband had a client who was an eye surgeon. Ironically, she was at the salon after I returned from my eye appointment. I was crying hysterically and didn't know what to do. She offered to meet with me the next day, which was a Sunday, and do a thorough examination of my eye. She thought a brain aneurysm diagnosis was premature and I needed further testing. Before I knew it, I was in a neurologist's office scheduling an MRI of my brain.

When I got the online report with the results from the testing, I was terrified. The MRI showed three suspicious spots on my brain. The radiologist said that one spot looked like a glioma (or tumor), one resembled an aneurysm, and the other a possible hemorrhage. The following day, I met with the neurologist, and he said that he called the radiologist because he didn't fully trust his assessment of my scan. He agreed that I had some suspicious spots, but he wasn't convinced that it was as grave as the report made it seem. I cannot even remotely express our relief. He recommended that I be monitored every six months to see if there were any changes.

Going through that experience has been one of my scariest health conditions to date. I got monitored every six months for two years to make sure none of the spots changed. I have to admit that any type of headache or even twitch in my head made me nervous for a few years. The neurologist believed the explosive headaches were triggered by hormones (you know how fun menopause can be), and that the spots may have been on my brain my entire life. It may have been a coincidence that they started when I tried that medication for the inflammation in my hands. There was no way of knowing. Having something wrong with my brain is another frightening thing that lurks in the back of my mind once in a while, but now that time has passed, I'm calmer about it. I'll live with some aches and pains, but I'm fucked if there is something wrong with my brain.

As I try to think positively about my head and go on with my life, I'm still having problems with my hands. I go back to the rheumatologist and talk to her again. This time she recommends that I start taking turmeric, the Indian spice. She explains that it can be a very effective anti-inflammatory. She also recommended some stretches and ice. Finding a doctor in the United States who believes in holistic medicine is such a gift. That was when I decided to go back to acupuncture on a more regular basis. To this day, I still have De Quervain's tenosynovitis, but it's manageable. I do have some carpal tunnel as well, but it's an occupational hazard that I have chosen to live with. I use my hands all day at my job. It is what it is.

In addition to the cranky bones and tendons, I've experienced a lot of gynecological pain throughout my lifetime. It started when I was a teenager. I found out pretty quickly that my body liked to produce cysts on my ovaries. When I would ovulate or menstruate, the cysts would often burst, and the pain would be indescribable. My mother would give me cough syrup with codeine to try to calm me down. Sometimes she would pull out the whiskey bottle if we were out of cough syrup. It was a pretty miserable indoctrination into womanhood. Fortunately, I discovered that being on the birth control pill lessened the number of cysts that my body produced.

Now, forty years later, I was still having pain in that area. As I approached that magical menopausal state, I hoped that things would be better in that part of my body. I guess I was being a bit too optimistic. I went for my yearly gynecological exam and asked my doctor for an ultrasound because I felt like I had a pretty big cyst on my left ovary and that something was growing in my uterus that shouldn't be there. He kindly agreed to let me have an ultrasound. Be careful what you ask for. It was a very painful exam, which was unusual. Normally, the transvaginal ultrasound test never bothered me. Things had changed. He said I did have a cyst on my ovary as I suspected. I also had several fibroids in my uterus—five to be exact. They were only two centimeters each, but if you add that up, it equals ten total. He said they were safe and shouldn't bother me. He thought it was remarkable that I knew a foreign object was invading my lady parts. Uh… hello? I feel EVERYTHING!

He told me that he wanted to order some blood work to see where I was with menopause. Between the hot flashes and mood swings, I had a nagging feeling that I knew what the blood work would say. Let's add insult to injury. Cysts…fibroids…and, oh yeah, old age on the horizon. Since I had an endometrial ablation when I was thirty-nine years old to combat periods that mirrored a crime scene every month, using my period as an indicator of menopause wasn't an option since I hadn't menstruated for over a decade. Now it was time to see what the blood works said. I could hardly wait.

I want to reiterate that I had the same gynecologist for over thirty years. I loved the guy. He was the one who basically told me that I needed to take a shit back when I was nineteen years old and to not worry about being infertile. Ultimately, he delivered all of our children and even performed several surgical procedures on me. I couldn't have asked for a better OBGYN, and I recommended him to countless clients over the years because I liked him that much. He passed away a few years ago at the tender age of sixty-seven and I was devastated. I even spoke at his celebration of life, because I was a huge fan and still miss him to this day.

Since I do Brazilian waxing for a living and have spent my career working with vaginas, my doctor and I had something in common. We shared stories and laughed a lot. It made all of my issues easier to cope with. He was an important part of my support system and I feel very grateful to have had him in my life.

There is one story in particular that makes me laugh every time I think about it. As I was walking into my kitchen after work one night, my cell phone rang. It was my gynecologist calling to tell me the results of my bloodwork. He told me that my blood tests showed that I had "graduated to the next stage." As he said that, my husband asked me who I was talking to. I told Mark who was on the phone and continued by telling him that the doctor just told me "I was freaking old!" The doctor overheard what I told Mark and assured me that he didn't say that. He had always tried to remain diplomatic in spite of my bizarre outbursts and random humor. I asked him what "graduating to the next stage" referred to. He tried to remain professional and said that the changes in my blood work explain the hormonal changes and discomfort I'd been experiencing. Was that supposed to make me feel better? Believe me, it didn't. I have hot flashes, random ovarian and uterine pain, and I don't even want to get into what's going on between my legs. Oh, I was going through some changes all right, and they weren't pleasing me. I reiterated to him the obvious fact that the bloodwork definitely showed I was getting old.

He offered me a few suggestions about hormone therapy, blah blah blah. I told him I'd think about his suggestions and thanked him for calling me. I ended up trying an estrogen device that got inserted into my vagina and left there. It was supposed to help with the Mojave Desert situation and the aging v-j-jay. That was a disaster. I can't deal with foreign parts in me; they hurt too much. It was time to go back to the drawing board. Hot flashes, fatigue, dryness, pain…welcome to my world. Like I don't have enough issues. I'm so glad that part of my life is over.

The next day I blogged about how disconcerting it was to find out that, not only do your bones deteriorate and clinically show how the aging process has affected your body, but so can your blood. My blood said I was getting older and in menopause. My response? "Menopause can kiss my ass!"

So, it appeared that my body was changing, and there were things that are completely out of my control. I didn't like that. I had done a pretty great job dealing with all the shit I've had to overcome, but getting older wasn't going to be one of them. At this point, the hot flashes had gotten worse, and I started to have more frequent fibro flare-ups again. It was more difficult keeping my weight stable and I seemed to be in a constant state of dehydration. Oh yeah, and I kept experiencing more injuries more easily than ever. But I continued to fight this thoroughly obnoxious aging process and continue to persevere. If you didn't notice by now, I'm a pretty determined gal and refuse to succumb fully to any problem that rears its ugly head.

But the problems kept coming. For example, when I started this part of the book, I was trying to recover from Achilles tendonitis from a racquetball injury. Even though I keep myself fit, within five minutes of playing racquetball, I felt something extremely unpleasant in my achilles. A few years ago, I played some pretty competitive racquetball several times a week. In addition, I actually played fairly well that day. Sadly, my body wasn't feeling it. The next thing I knew, I was wearing one of those sexy boots for two weeks.

Six months passed and I was still struggling with a pissed-off Achilles. It took forever to heal. The upside is that I didn't need surgery and didn't have to miss any work. If I had to sit around and recover from another surgery, you may have had to send me to the psych ward.

If it isn't one thing, it's another. My body just seems to be fragile, and things keep happening no matter how hard I try to protect myself. It is important for every one of us to keep up with our health, and I feel like I'm constantly struggling to be and feel as good as humanly possible. It's frustrating, but it's how it is. I just remind myself that wallowing isn't productive and won't make me happy. In fact, it makes the feeling so much worse. For those of you with some funky ailment, I can totally understand when it becomes overwhelming, but I also want to encourage you to try to persevere and find things in your life that bring you joy. I know I say that a lot, but I really mean it.

It probably won't surprise you that there is more annoying shit that has happened since the neck, knee, brain, hands, lady parts, and Achilles... Isn't that a surprise? At forty-seven, I went to the plastic surgeon because I had two TINY spots on each temple that would bleed periodically. They were small, red, and perfectly round. That was it—nothing spectacular. They didn't hurt or look strange, but they would randomly bleed without warning. One of the spots had been there for a year, and I didn't get thoroughly annoyed until I had one on either side of my face. When they both would bleed at the same time, I felt like a freak.

When the doctor (my plastic surgeon) looked at my face, he shook his head and politely scolded me for not coming in as soon as they appeared (about a year prior). He told me they were a form of skin cancer called basal cell carcinoma. I knew what that was, and I also knew it wasn't something that I wanted. I adamantly told him I was too young to have skin cancer and didn't want basal cell. He laughed and said he was sorry but that was what I had. He told me that whenever I found a mole that bleeds, it is very likely cancer, and I needed to get in to see him right away. On top of everything else, now I had skin cancer? WTF!

He quickly removed them and put a tiny stitch in each area to close them up. It was impressive because I didn't feel anything and couldn't find any scars from where he did it. That is why I go to a plastic surgeon for these kinds of procedures. While he was examining the rest of my face, he noticed a patch of dry skin on the right side of my cheek that he wanted to biopsy because he told me that it looked suspicious. He asked me how long the patch had been there, and to be honest, I had no idea. I never really paid attention to it since I just thought it was a patch of dry skin. His office called me a few days later to schedule a surgical procedure to have the spot removed. I really thought it was dry skin, which is something I deal with on a regular basis. I guess it was something more, but for some reason, I wasn't worried about it.

Mark went with me to the appointment because he loves watching any kind of surgical procedure. They said it would take less than an hour, so I booked two hours off from work in the middle of the day to get it removed. First, he numbed practically the entire left side of my face, which was a really creepy feeling. Next, I felt a lot of pressure on my cheek. I asked Mark, "Did he just *Silence of the Lambs* my face?"

Mark looked at the area and said, "Yeah, he did." Then he asked the surgeon why he "*Silence of the Lamb*ed my face." I immediately started to cry. Mark asked me if it hurt. I told him it didn't; the idea of it just freaked me out. I couldn't stop the tears from flowing, and although I was trying to be brave, the sensation of him cutting open my face was really creepy. The doctor said that it was a fairly large tumor and he wanted to make sure he got it all out. Tumor? What the hell! They took thirty margins of skin out, and diagnosed them as having squamous cell carcinoma—another form of skin cancer. I couldn't believe it. Now I had two types of skin cancer. Thankfully he got it all, even though I have a fairly large scar on my left cheek.

Vanity kind of goes out the window when things like this happen. Yes, I have a pretty decent-sized scar on the left side of my face. But, if left untreated, my face could have been deformed because it would have continued to spread. That would have really sucked. So, I'm grateful he found it, and I try to think of my scar as a badass kind of look. I've never been in a fight, so this is as close as I'll probably ever get to looking like I was in a bar room brawl.

The following year I got a tattoo on my thigh. The tattoo was the logo from my third book entitled *The Happy Trail*. It is the outline of a curvaceous woman's body with a pair of lips imprinted on the ass. It was my fifth tattoo, but it was the first one that had colored ink on it. Although the lips on my trademarked logo are hot pink, I had them tattooed in red. Apparently, red can act as a carcinogen (how the hell was I supposed to know that?). I got the tattoo in November, noticed a funky multi-colored bump growing out of the lips in December, and had it removed at the beginning of February. When he was making the incision, I felt a lot of pressure on my thigh. I asked Mark (he was there again, of course) if the doctor was digging to China because that is what it felt like. Mark looked at how deep the incision was and just said, "Yep." When he asked the surgeon why he was cutting so deep, he said the tumor had roots. How special is that? My skin is now like a vegetable garden that is growing mysterious things with roots. As it turned out, the bump was another cancerous tumor, which he suspected was exasperated by the red ink. I just couldn't catch a break. While he was stitching up the incision, I asked him what the lips on the tattoo were going to look like. He stepped back, looked at it for a second, and said, "Thin."

Now, I've been dealing with several forms of skin cancer on random parts of my body for a few years. Up to this point, none of the tumors I've had removed have been melanoma, so I've felt blessed by that fact. That's the scary one. I read an article that said more people die from melanoma than any other type of cancer in the United States. I also remember one of the dermatologists I went to said that even if I have basal and squamous cell cancers, that doesn't mean that I will necessarily get melanoma. That was relieving to hear after all of the people I have met who have had loved one's die from the disease. So now I go for regular checkups, every four to six months, keep my skin mostly out of the sun, and check it on a regular basis.

Unfortunately, everything changed in December of 2018.

I went to get a full body check by the dermatologist's physician assistant right before Christmas. I like her better than the actual doctor at the facility because she is much more thorough and seems to actually care about my skin and about me. The owner of the facility spent a whopping six minutes with me during the previous visit and missed two squamous cells, which I had my plastic surgeon remove later that month, so now I stick with the PA. As a side note, I have been to many different dermatologists over the years and have been disappointed with their lack of empathy and lackadaisical approach to getting a full body scan. You would be shocked how difficult it is to find someone who is thorough and actually gives a shit about my sun-damaged, old-lady skin. It's also incredible how blasé most of them are about the fact that I have skin cancer, even if it isn't the fatal kind. In addition, they all seem to be so busy that they do a half-assed job checking the body and move on to the next hunk of skin. It has been disheartening, to say the least. Anyway, as the PA was checking me, she blew right by a small spot on my thigh that looked a little creepy to me. I made her go back and look at it again. She asked me if the spot was new. How the hell was I supposed to know? I have a lot of skin and it has a multitude of freckles, old age spots, and all sorts of ugly-looking splotches on it. It seemed creepy since it was black and had an irregular shape. I told her that it was darker than most of my freckles and that it "looked funky." She wasn't sold on the fact it could be bad, but she appeased me by taking a biopsy. It was frustrating because she's the expert, not me. I always check my skin as thoroughly as possible before my appointments, but I have a lot of surface area, and a lot of weird-colored spots on my body. I can't even see a lot of my skin because it's behind me!

She actually took four biopsies, and a few days later, a nurse from their office called me. The nurse casually told me that the spot on the outside of my left leg was squamous, the spot on my left calf was fine, the spot on my right thigh was melanoma, and the spot on my right tricep was fine. Wait. What? She couldn't have been more matter of fact and unemotional. She might as well have been dictating to me her fucking grocery list by the way she was reading through my laundry list of spots. I immediately started to sob. "Oh, you're upset?" she said. Are you kidding me? What is wrong with people?

"Yes, I'm upset. Do you know how many people die from melanoma?" I choked.

"Um, well… Do you want the NP to call you?" I felt like I was in the *Twilight Zone* with this conversation.

"No," was all I said. She told me that since it was melanoma, I needed to go to a plastic surgeon as soon as possible to have it removed.

I felt like I was punched in the stomach. I was at work and completely broke down. When I was sort of able to breathe, I called my husband and told them what they said. I also told him he should have kicked the tires a lot harder before he married me because I was a fucking mess. We went to the surgeon that night, and he assured me it was stage zero, and after the holidays were over and my skin had healed, he would remove it. I was relieved it was centralized in my epidermis, but I was, and still am, completely freaked out. I loved loved *loved* the sun, and I couldn't believe that it led to this. I currently alternate between the dermatologist and the plastic surgeon every two to three months so that I have two separate sets of eyes checking me out.

This is now my new normal, getting my skin checked regularly. It takes time and costs money, but I don't have a choice. If I don't keep on top of it, it could turn into something more serious and even fatal. Just another thing on my list…

Aside from getting things burned or cut off over the years, I have used a topical chemotherapy treatment on my face, neck, and thigh. It burns the skin like a strong facial peel and then brings a lot of cancer to the surface so it can be removed. The lotion has more side effects than just burning, itching, and bleeding skin, however. I swear the treatment affects me systemically and makes me experience chemo-like symptoms. When I would use it at night, I would wake up in the morning nauseous, dizzy, and achy. After several applications, I would develop open sores on my skin that were so painful, I couldn't handle the water hitting them in the shower. I ultimately gave up on it because I couldn't handle how sickly it made me feel and how gross my face and chest looked with open wounds on them.

Fibro patients are sensitive to a myriad of things, and it always astounds me when I talk to other people who suffer from the same strange sensitivities that I do. For example, I have problems with bright lights. Driving on a sunny day when there is snow on the ground is a huge issue for me. One day, I actually had to pull over to the side of the road and switch places with my husband because my eyes were tearing and burning so badly from the sunlight that I couldn't drive. Ironically, I was recently waxing a woman who was diagnosed with fibro, and she complained that the lights in my wax room were too bright, making her feel sick. I'm happy to say I came up with a solution to that problem; she wears sunglasses during the service now.

I'm also hypersensitive to cold. When I get really cold, I often feel like crying because it is so painful. It's not just that I get goosebumps and shake like a normal person would react to being chilly. I feel it so much deeper than that. It's as if the cold is constricting my bones in the most bizarre way. It's very uncomfortable and sometimes unbearable.

I'm also sensitive to smells. I'd like to chop my husband's head off every time he uses Febreze in the house or at work. It seriously makes me want to hurt someone. Many cleaning solutions, perfumes, and other artificial smells are irritating as well. I like to stick to the smell of homemade cooking, like the smell of garlic or lemon. I haven't worn cologne in decades because the smell makes me physically ill.

Sometimes my skin hurts. I have joint pain, nerve pain, and basically all-over pain. I get weak, tired, and sometimes confused. The multitude of annoying responses I experience are just something that I've had to learn to deal with and I've tried to deal with them with as much dignity and positivity as possible. If you create some kind of mantra that reminds you to focus on the positive and try to make every day count, you will have an easier time accepting the cards that have been dealt to you.

As you can see, I've had a ton of shit to deal with over the years, but my fight continues because I cannot and will not let it win. I have three amazing kids that I know will want to get married one day, and they all have expressed the desire to have children of their own. In fact, since I started this book, my oldest got married and had a baby. Believe me, I intend on being here for them as long as possible and enjoying them every step of the way.

CHAPTER 8

VITAMINS GALORE

My husband and I own a couple of busy beauty salons and interact with a ton of people every week. Whenever the topic of autoimmune diseases comes up, I often share that I'm a fibro sufferer. I don't do it for sympathy or pity. On the contrary, I like to inspire women (since most fibro patients are women) and offer suggestions that could potentially help them live a more fulfilling life.

I have many clients who are anxious to hear what kind of supplements I take since I don't take any prescription medications. It's not an easy question to answer, because I have tried a multitude of different things over the years, and it has been difficult to pinpoint which ones really do any good or make any kind of difference. I most definitely know which ones I need to stay away from, however, and that realization is worth talking about. In addition, I'm constantly mixing up what I take depending on my symptoms, the time of year, and often just my mood at the moment. And boy can I be moody sometimes.

Let's start with the good ol' multivitamin. Since the majority of vitamins produced in our country are synthetic, their efficacy is minimal at best. Our bodies weren't designed to absorb synthetic products, so the majority of the benefits pass through us when we urinate. That alone is a good enough reason to not waste your money on them. If I did decide to try a multivitamin again, it would be completely natural and organic and have a lot of studies that support its efficacy. Now that I think about it, I haven't taken a multi in decades because they have always given me a terrible stomachache. Although I generally do not experience stomach problems, taking a multivitamin is one way to make sure I feel sick. And, believe me, I have tried a plethora of multivitamins over the years and have never felt anything but sick. Feeling shitty is reason enough for me to ditch them. Many health practitioners will encourage you to get your vitamins through your diet. I like that idea a whole lot more.

Since I've gone through menopause, and my bone density has decreased a little bit, my health practitioners keep drilling me about taking calcium. I appreciate their diligence in keeping my bones nice and strong, but calcium has the same effect on me that a multivitamin does; it wrecks my stomach. I have tried a variety of calcium supplements and all of them make me feel nauseous. It's not worth it to me. Once again, I prefer to get calcium the old-fashioned way—through my diet. Calcium can be found in leafy green vegetables like spinach and kale, soybeans, white beans, and even salmon. I would rather have baked salmon over spinach any day of the week over a calcium pill that makes me feel like I have morning sickness. I was okay with morning sickness when I was pregnant, but any other time isn't worth it.

I've taken chewable vitamin C tablets for years, even though I think I get a decent amount of C in my diet. Most people assume that vitamin C only exists in fruit, but it can be found in other types of food as well. Personally, I don't eat a lot of fruit because I am prone to sores in my mouth. I have discovered that acidic foods will create painful sores in my mouth and on my tongue, which is a clear sign to me that I shouldn't ingest them. Once again, it's all about listening to your body. Have you started listening yet?

If I do eat fruit, it is always in small quantities, and it has to be at room temperature. For as long as I can remember, cold fruit hurts my teeth. I think vitamin C is crucial in our diet, and we are lucky that we can get it in other foods as well. Broccoli and Brussels sprouts are two excellent sources of the vitamin. There is also vitamin C in parsley and lemons, which are the main ingredients in tabouli and a salad that I like to make. Tabouli is a Lebanese bulgur salad that I often make for my family because it is fresh, extremely nutritious, and delicious. It is spectacular how many different vitamins exist in food, and if you do your homework, you should be able to supplement where you are deficient through your meal planning.

When I was growing up, I remember my father and my grandfather taking some really smelly vitamin B tablets. They were both pretty healthy guys and swore by this vitamin. I have tried a variety of B vitamins over the years and have never been wowed by any of them. I wish I knew what kind they took. Research claims that B deficiencies can cause depression, confusion, and even weakened immune systems. That's a scary thought. Although there are many benefits to taking B vitamins, you must make sure you take a good brand. I try to stay away from cheap, low-quality brands of vitamins. I think it's better to get your nutrients through your diet before you waste your time on a vitamin that may serve little purpose. B vitamins are also supposed to help with hormones and metabolism, so I continue to take them because I've been feeling pretty good, and I'd prefer not to rock my shaky boat.

I get my vitamin D levels tested every year, and it tends to be on the low side unless I take a five-thousand-milligram supplement on a daily basis—and even then, it tends to be low. I live in one of the cloudiest cities in the country, so I am not alone in my need to absorb more D in my system. Rochester, New York, is known for having a population that is deficient in this. They say one of the best ways to absorb this vitamin is through the sun, but, as you now know, I can't enjoy the sun as much anymore. So, I rely on a little pill.

Vitamin D can also be found in tuna and salmon, which I try to eat weekly. If you're a sushi lover like I am, and need an excuse to eat sushi more regularly, since it can be expensive, chalk it up to a vitamin deficiency and feel better about the expense.

Vitamin D also exists in many foods and drinks that I don't typically enjoy, however, such as orange juice, soymilk, cereal, and beef liver. I only drink orange juice if it's freshly squeezed, which I am lucky I can get at my local grocery store. Once again, it's expensive, but if I want a mimosa, this is the only way to go. All other orange juices that you find in the grocery store bother my system and I don't like how they taste. There is a fair amount of research that has discovered our society drinks too much juice that is filled with a ton of sugar and other additives that just aren't good for you. I know that freshly squeezed can be expensive, but there are other options. What about eating an orange instead? It's such a better option and so much better for you.

The only time I use a milk product is in my morning protein shakes. I don't drink milk anymore, because the dairy bothers my digestive system. As far as alternative milk products, I'm not a fan of the taste of soymilk, and I have tried many different kinds over the years. I tend to use almond, coconut, or cashew milk in my shakes. There are a variety of blends of the three that I just mentioned that I like as well. I'm thrilled that we now have so many choices of milk that don't come from cows.

Since cereal has gluten in it, I tend to avoid eating it. Besides, I'm pretty convinced that most cereals have little nutritional benefits in them. If I do have a bowl of cereal, I am never satiated. That alone tells me something. But the hard-to-pronounce ingredients on the side of the box are what really turn me off. All of the cereals that are made of fake sweeteners or ingredients such as marshmallows or candies make no sense to me at all. In my mind, most cereals equate to junk food. Why not just have a piece of cake for breakfast? At least there might be an egg in it to give you a little nutritional value to it. I know there are some cereals that have more nutritional value than others, but I still shy away from them. None of the members in my immediate family are cereal eaters either because they weren't raised eating it. My kids were more likely to have eggs or a slice of pizza for breakfast. I made the conscientious decision to not have cereal be a staple for my children in the morning. I noticed when the sugar high subsided, they'd crash hard, and that could make it difficult for them to concentrate when they were in school. I was conscientious about providing more nutritional options for my kids, and you should be too. You'll never convince me that Pop-Tarts are a good choice of nutrition for your kids in the morning.

I have taken vitamin E periodically as an adult. It's supposed to help with your skin, and since I have a lot of wrinkles and skin cancer, it sounds like a viable supplement to take. A few years ago, I read an article that said that the combination of evening primrose oil (which can be good for skin, hormones, and arthritis) and vitamin E can help with menopause symptoms.

Since I've been struggling for several years with menopause and hot flashes, I took the combination for a few years. At the time I wasn't sure how much it helped or not, but I survived menopause fairly gracefully so I think it may have done some good.

Fish oil is another supplement that I know a lot of people take, including me. There's a lot of research about all the amazing benefits of taking fish oil. It can help your heart, increase brain and eye function, reduce inflammation, help improve your skin, help women in pregnancy and while breastfeeding, reduce liver fat, and the list continues. The problem that I find is deciding which fish oil to take. There are a variety of different types of fish oils on the market and it is confusing to make a decision on which one to take. Sometimes too many choices are daunting. If your research cannot help you decide, I'd ask a nutritionist. I take different ones to mix it up because everyone has a different opinion about which one is the best for you. One month it may be cod liver, the next month it may be something else. I get bored taking the same thing unless I feel confident that it is making a difference, so this is one supplement I mix up.

My mother turned ninety-three years old this year. She still works, has two dogs, drives a fancy sports car, lives with a man twenty-seven years her junior, and takes **ZERO** medication. She had a knee replacement a few years ago and has some arthritis but is generally in excellent health. When she was growing up, her father used to give her a large spoonful of cod liver oil every morning. She is convinced that that has something to do with her good health all these years, in addition to not taking any prescription medication. I pray that I follow in this amazing woman's footsteps.

The jury is still out on turmeric supplements as far as I'm concerned. Thus far, they have had little effect in reducing the inflammation in my hands. However, it's hard to make a clear judgement on them since I continue to piss my hands off due to the type of job I have. I have found that when I ingest turmeric supplements as a tea, I feel a little less achy and swollen. That alone is worth it. I have bought turmeric tea bags, but the powder seems to be the most effective. My concoction is as follows: one teaspoon of powdered turmeric, one tea bag (black tea in the afternoon for a pick-me-up or herbal tea in the evening), five whole peppercorns, and a tablespoon of organic, dark maple syrup. The peppercorns are supposed to activate the curcumin in the turmeric, which is the active ingredient that is supposed to help with inflammation. The tea bag adds flavor, caffeine, or other benefits depending on what flavor you choose. The maple syrup has a lot of nutrients in it and makes the tea more pleasant to drink. Even if it doesn't result in an obvious, external reduction in inflammation, I'm pretty convinced it reduces some inflammation deep inside me, and that lessens my discomfort. I need to give you the downside of drinking powdered turmeric, however. The first time I finished a mug of tea, I left work to go to the bank. When I looked in the rear-view mirror to put on lipstick, I realized I had orange teeth! It was so disgusting looking. Whenever I tell people about my homemade tea remedy, I also tell them that it is imperative that they brush their teeth when they finish or they'll look like they sucked on a pumpkin, too.

My acupuncturist recommended I start taking an organic iron supplement because my blood seemed stagnant to her. Even though I eat a lot of iron-rich foods like tofu, broccoli, dark chocolate, and spinach, she felt that some of my exhaustion, dangerously low blood pressure, and poor circulation were due to an iron deficiency. If it could help my lousy sleep patterns, then it was worth a try. The fibro symptoms that interrupt me at night in addition to the hot flashes from menopause have made my search for REM sleep worse than finding the proverbial needle in a haystack. I alternate between waking up every hour or two to waking up at two thirty in the morning and staring at the clock until the sun rises. Even though this kind of sleep pattern has been going on for years, I've never felt the kind of exhaustion that I've felt in the last year. There have been times when I feared that I was suffering from chronic fatigue syndrome, which is a common caveat of fibromyalgia sufferers. To be honest, I probably have that as well, but I really cannot deal with one more disease, condition, or syndrome attached to my name. I fight my fatigue with as much gusto as I can muster. When the exhaustion became more pronounced, I knew I needed something to help. I've felt a little better since I started taking the iron.

I briefly commented on my blood pressure, but I should share more with you in case you can relate. I have always had low blood pressure. Anything over 90/60 makes me feel like I am having a heart attack. (I know, Drama Queen strikes again). One day, I went to our local pain clinic to discuss my completely fucked up neck. When the nurse took my blood pressure, she actually smacked the machine and wondered why my numbers weren't registering. I had a feeling why. My blood pressure was 75/45. As she wrote down the results, she asked me if I got dizzy. I told her that as I was walking into the facility, I sneezed and not only did it cause stabbing pain in my neck, I also felt a dizzy sensation in my head. I figured my pressure was low that morning. Since I have always suffered from low blood pressure, I was used to it and didn't really put much thought into it until she smacked the machine. I knew I felt lightheaded and basically goofy in the head that particular morning, but it is a feeling that I experience on a fairly regular basis. It's interesting how our minds can adjust to the negative changes in our body and learn to adapt to the symptoms, like being dizzy. It's almost as if being dizzy is just another normal and I barely notice it unless the conversation comes up.

It's funny how some people can have low blood pressure and feel absolutely fine. When mine gets below 90/60, I can tell. My body feels strange—often shaky and cold. My head also feels strange, and I tend to get dizzy if I pick up something from the floor or move too quickly. I believe that fibro patients are more sensitive to changes in their bodies. Weird changes, like my dizzy brain, are conditions that I need to embrace, as I can't always control them. If you have a weird thing that happens to you, I suggest you try to be more accepting. It is possible that you may or may not be able to change it or have the kind of control over it that you may want. But you can learn to adapt. When I'm feeling lightheaded, I drink more water and am more conscientious about my movements. Sometimes I reach for the pickle or pepperoncini jar. They help as well. I am confident that you have the ability to help yourself feel better if you put your mind to it. I have to laugh because one time a doctor suggested I add more salt to my diet to help with my blood pressure. So now one of the things I have changed is that I no longer ask the bartender to hold the salt when I order a margarita.

I feel very strongly that you need to choose your vitamin supplements carefully. Too many pills, herbs, vitamins, or supplements can cause adverse effects that can ultimately make you feel a lot worse. Pay attention to what you put in your mouth. Keep a journal. Listen to your body. And remember, just because calcium doesn't work for me doesn't mean that you won't be able to take it with zero negative reactions. Everyone's body is unique, and you need to pay attention to what does—and what does not—make you feel better or give you some relief.

CHAPTER 9

COFFEE, TEA, OR M.E.?

The first thing I do every morning is have a cup of coffee. I don't sleep well, and the caffeine helps get me going. It also gets my bowels going, which is important. My husband usually goes downstairs to make it and brings it upstairs to me, because I have a really hard time walking down the stairs first thing in the morning. If I don't take one step at a time, I worry about my knees collapsing. I also struggle with foot pain, so it takes a little while to get the circulation going.

There are known benefits to drinking coffee, so I don't worry about having it every day. Research claims coffee consumption can lower the risk of Alzheimer's, diabetes, heart disease, stroke, cancer, liver disease, and even Parkinson's. I think adding a ton of sugary additives negates many of the benefits, but I have no qualms about having a cup when I wake up since I only add a little bit of cream to it. Now that I think of it, is it even called waking up if you stay up the entire night?

I also like tea, just not first thing in the morning. We sure are creatures of habit, aren't we? I have to be careful what kind of tea I drink, however. I can only drink green tea if it isn't very strong. For some reason, the caffeine in green tea makes my heart palpitate and gives me a nauseous stomach. Licorice tea is a definite no-no. Licorice has the ability to naturally detoxify your system. Apparently, my body doesn't like to detoxify. When I have too much, I see bizarre spots in front of my eyes. It also makes me nauseated.

Peppermint is supposed to be good for the system, especially digestion, but it makes me flushed and queasy. Chamomile does the same thing. I tend to drink pretty basic black tea, not too strong. If you keep a journal of when you eat or drink something that makes you feel crappy, you will find a pattern. We are more sensitive than the average Joe, so it's important to establish what specifically adds to your misery or your discomfort. By the way, have you purchased your blank journal yet, or do you plan to keep notes on your phone?

Have you ever heard the expression "sow your wild oats?" If not, I have something interesting to share with you. Oat straw is part of the same plant that oatmeal comes from. In the Middle Ages, people believed that oat straw could help with cognition. In more recent times, oat straw is believed to help with circulation and can also act as a sexual enhancement supplement. Other research suggests that oat straw can help with depression and mood. Since those suffering from fibro often have circulatory issues, low sex drive, and depression, oat straw can be beneficial. I bought my first bag of oat straw from a health food store. Now I order it online because it's more cost-effective. I boil the straw in water and then let it steep for a few hours. Drinking it makes me feel good, and it doesn't give me any of the negative side effects that some teas give me. Since I get dehydrated easily, consuming unsweetened and non-carbonated liquids is important. Maybe oat straw is something that you'd like to try out.

As I said earlier, I don't drink any juice unless it is freshly squeezed. I can't consume most juices, because added sugars and flavoring don't agree with me. Drinks made from concentrate or that have anything artificial in them are not a good idea for anyone. There is too much artificial crap in our foods and drinks, and we need to stay away from them and steer our kids away from them also. I mostly drink water throughout the day, because I can pronounce every ingredient on the label, so I don't have to worry about having some kind of weird negative reaction. And I usually have tea in the afternoons, often with a large hunk of lemon. Sometimes I mix my oat straw with black tea so there is a little caffeine boost. Be careful if you drink a lot of tea, however, because it can stain your teeth.

This is a random story that still cracks me up and I have to share. One time, a woman asked me how old I was. When I told her I was fifty, she said she couldn't believe it. I said thank you to her. "Do you want to know why you don't look fifty years old?" she asked.

"Sure," I said. She told me that most women start to look old because their teeth get yellow, and they don't have eyelashes. I told her I brush my teeth four to five times a day and use a lash enhancement serum on my lashes. I thought it was a funny thing for her to say. Since when are lashes and teeth the defining factor of age? I do combat discolored teeth with a little baking soda mixed with my toothpaste now and again because I'd prefer not to have yellow teeth either. And I'm psyched that lash extensions and lash serums have become so popular because they make me feel prettier, too. As long as I didn't look my age, I was happy.

Carbonated beverages are another substance that can aggravate your digestive system. For one thing, carbonation can cause bloating and gas. I don't partake in anything that can cause me to toot or look unnaturally pregnant. Neither of those conditions are inherently sexy. C'mon, who doesn't like to feel sexy? Carbonation is also acidic, and I have learned that acidic products are detrimental to how I feel. The acidity can also lead to calcium and magnesium loss, which are things you want to avoid. Low magnesium levels can lead to fatigue, muscle cramps, and restless leg syndrome. Basically, if you pay attention to how you feel, then drinking a Pepsi will probably make you feel shitty, and you need to decide if it is really worth it. If you feel you can't live without soda every day, you need to assess your addiction to sugar.

When my night sweats began, I started getting a lot more light-headed when I worked out in the morning. I tried eating before I went to the gym, but I'd get nauseous and that was totally counter-productive. Then I discovered a product called Xtend® BCAA'S. Several companies make similar products to this one. This just happens to be the one that I add to my water. I've also used Blox from GNC, and that seems to do the same thing. I mix one scoop in my water bottle when I go to the gym. It helps to replenish electrolytes, which is important when you sweat a lot. For me, it prevents me from getting dizzy and helps me stay hydrated. I usually have a second scoop with a large bottle of water that I take to work and try to consume by noon. The company claims it supports muscle growth and recovery. All I know is that it's tastier than regular water, which makes it easier to consume larger quantities, and I feel better when I drink it. I've even used it as a mixer with vodka and ice as a refreshing summer drink. Well, now I sound like a commercial for them. They really should hire me to sell their product. Regardless, hydration is key, and whatever helps you drink a lot of water can only make you feel better. When I function in a dehydrated state, I'm also more prone to urinary tract infections, and that is never a good time.

Aloe juice can also be an excellent source of hydration for you. Personally, I have a difficult time drinking it. There is something about the consistency that bothers me. I have been more successful using coconut water in my shakes in the morning, because that is also an excellent source of hydration and easier to digest than milk products.

I cannot stress enough how important it is to pay attention to what goes in your mouth, even if it's a liquid. Many people ignore the drinks that they ingest as contributors to their aches and pains. Liquids count too. I know I'm getting to sound like a broken record, but you need to be more aware of the cause and effect of external foods, sounds, smells, and the like. If you can pinpoint even just a few triggers, you will feel better.

CHAPTER 10

SUCKY SURGERIES AND PETULANT PROCEDURES

firmly believe that any kind of trauma, whether positive or negative, can intensify our pain and disrupt our fragile systems. I've had a lot of surgical procedures over the years, and writing this book has forced me to go back in time and reflect on the circumstances surrounding some of them. What I realized was that any type of change that occurs in my body tends to elicit heightened sensations that "normal" people would probably not experience.

One summer, my husband and I were at a cousin's party in a local park. I was sitting in a fold-up chair talking to some of the ladies. Mark brought me over a bottle of Corona. I took a sip of beer and rested the bottle on my stomach. I felt a really weird pain in my stomach from the weight of the bottle. I knew it only weighed about a pound, but it felt a lot heavier than that. When I felt my stomach with my hand, it felt really tender. It was on the right side near my waist.

The next morning, my stomach still felt a little distended and tender. I went to my internist, and he ordered a CAT scan. The doctor told me to refrain from eating in case I needed surgery. The next day I was sent to a general surgeon to review the scan. It was a weird encounter I'll never forget. It was a Tuesday, and I had an appointment with him first thing in the morning before I was scheduled to go to work. I always dress up for work and make sure my hair and makeup are done. When he walked into the room, he scanned me from top to bottom. His assessment of my physicality was deliberate and made me feel uncomfortable. "Why are you here?" he asked with impatience, like he suspected I was wasting his precious time. It was obvious his bedside manner sucked, and I felt an instantaneous dislike for this man.

"Because my stomach is sore and distended," I told him.

"Well, you look fine," he said. Okay, this guy was an ass and I wanted to slap him.

"I am fine as long as you don't touch my stomach," I told him matter-of-factly and a little snotty. He told me he reviewed the CAT scan, and it was inconclusive.

He doubted anything was wrong with me.

He asked me to lie on the table. When he pressed down on the lower right part of my stomach, I couldn't believe how much it hurt. I grabbed his arm tightly to pull it away from my body and growled, "I told you not to press on my stomach." The way he pressed on my stomach was the way they always test for appendicitis. It was like a quick jump on my lower side, and it was really painful.

He told me I probably needed it out even though the CAT scan was inconclusive because the physical test of jumping on my stomach was usually pretty accurate. I can't say I had much faith in the guy, but I didn't want my appendix to burst, so I agreed to go have the surgery. I went home and grabbed my husband so he could take me to the hospital. After the surgery, he told me my appendix looked fine, but I had a few cysts on my ovaries, which could have mimicked appendicitis pain. Although I knew I'd been cystic for years, I was pretty confident the pain wasn't from the cysts.

Five days after surgery, my husband and I had our annual summer party. It was always a big shindig, with roughly 150 people attending. We always had a bartender, a bounce house, and a ton of food. I was walking around gingerly since I had just had surgery. One of the attorney/soccer dads came up to me and asked me how I was feeling as he heard I had my appendix out that week. I told him that I was fine (of course I did) and that a little surgery wouldn't stop us from having the party. He asked me who did the surgery, so I told him his name. Apparently, he played golf with the surgeon on a regular basis. I told him that I thought his friend was an ass because he didn't take me seriously because I "looked good." He told me to tell him we were friends. I felt like it didn't matter at this point because the surgery was over, but I thought I'd drop his name for shits and giggles and see how the doctor responded.

The next day, I went for my follow-up. The first thing I said to him was that we had a mutual friend in common. All of a sudden, his demeanor completely changed. I try to treat everyone with kindness and respect no matter who they are, so his change in attitude actually pissed me off even more, but I also know how to play the game, so I went with it. Once our pleasantries passed, he said that he was shocked by the results of the biopsy. Apparently, the pathology showed that I did in fact have appendicitis. It was in the early stages, but it was indeed infected and needed to come out. He told me he was shocked I was able to detect the infection at such a premature stage. I told him I was very in tune with my body and always knew when something was wrong. I guess that's a good thing about having fibro—we are super sensitive to any changes in our bodies as long as we pay attention and listen to what our body is trying to tell us. I was glad I got it early on, so it didn't erupt during an inopportune moment, like when I was traveling and didn't have access to a hospital. I still wasn't a fan of the surgeon, but I was glad it was over.

A few weeks later, I went for a follow-up with my regular doctor because I was still having a decent amount of pain in the area. They said that the scar tissue around the site must have been what was bothering me. He said that most people don't feel sensitivity to the site a few weeks after the procedure but that it would pass in time. He didn't realize that fibro patients feel everything!

A few years went by, and I couldn't take how debilitating my periods were, so I decided to do something about it. I had an elective female surgery, called an endometrial ablation. I endured the surgery well and was able to return to work after a few days. In case you were wondering, an ablation is a surgical procedure that removes the entire uterine lining. This makes it so a woman never has to have a period again. Women often experience difficult and heavy menstrual cycles after they have a baby, and I was most definitely one of those women. Cutting the "monthly shark attack" from my life was definitely a blessing.

Even though I recovered well from the procedure, it was still traumatic to my body.

Every surgery and every procedure I have had, whether elective or not, causes stress on my body. The continued trauma wreaks havoc on our sensitive symptoms and makes a pain-free body nearly impossible.

The dentist is another place that I dread because it is a place where I always suffer. A routine cleaning can leave me sore for days. I tend to be a polite bitch when I go to the dentist because I feel like I always have to explain myself. For starters, I almost always refuse X-rays. I have three reasons for declining: One, it's expensive. Two, I don't want the radiation transmitted to me from X-rays since I'm paranoid about getting cancer and I've had way too many X-rays over the years. Three, I can't tolerate sticking the apparatus in my mouth. It hurts and leaves my mouth raw for days. But when I need something surgically done, then I know I'm in trouble. One time, I needed a root canal. Sadly, I learned during that procedure that I couldn't tolerate regular Novocain because it makes my heart race like crazy. Once you've suffered from anxiety, you avoid the heart-racing sensation at any cost. Apparently, there is an ingredient in Novocain called epinephrine that stimulates your heart, and it's something I try to avoid.

A few years later I clenched my teeth so hard during a head MRI, I broke a molar. They said it was an open MRI, which was bullshit. I'm legitimately claustrophobic and I felt like the white cream sandwiched between the two chocolate halves of an Oreo cookie with my head locked in a freaky football helmet contraption. It completely and utterly freaked me out. When I went to the dentist, I told her that I couldn't tolerate the epinephrine in the Novocain. She told me there was an alternative that wasn't quite as effective. I agreed to try it. What I quickly learned was that the numbing agent that doesn't contain the stimulating drug sucks, sucks big time. It doesn't numb the area as effectively, and it definitely doesn't penetrate to the root. My tongue was numb but that was about it. My regular dentist was out of town, so his associate had to grind the remainder of my tooth down to almost nothing. She kept hitting my nerves, which hurt like hell, but I didn't care. I didn't want the stronger numbing agent because it caused my heart to race, and I HATE when that happens.

She kept stopping to ask if I was all right. "Listen, I live in chronic pain. I can handle this. I also wax my own Brazilian. Just finish and stop asking me how I am. I'm fine!" It was a very tense exchange, and I just wanted it over. She became one of my least favorite dentists.

When I went back to get my fake tooth put in, also known as a crown, my husband called the dentist's office to see if I was okay. My regular dentist, who is a friend of the family, was surprised Mark was so worried about me. Mark knew how traumatizing dental procedures were to me and also knew how shitty my last visit to the dentist was. Our friend didn't realize how upsetting my last appointment was and felt bad that I was so stressed out about getting the tooth finished. I know it's hard for health practitioners to understand how fragile we can be, but we are hypersensitive to a lot of things. It's just how we are. We don't need your pity, just your understanding.

I truly believe in the importance of educating yourself. Haven't you heard the old adage that knowledge is power? I believe it is. Every time something bad happens to one of my body parts, I do my homework. When my knee blew up, and I was diagnosed with PVNS, I read every article I could find on the subject. I had a funky disease in the synovial fluid on my knee. Having the orthopedic surgeon give me a diagnosis and explain the surgery and all of its risks was not enough. I always need to know more. That is how I cope. Knowledge is indeed power, and I always need to know as much as possible about every injury or ailment that plagues me.

Feigning ignorance is never a good idea, so stop burying your head in the sand, because it isn't helping you at all. Take control of your health.

I also believe that knowledge gives you the control you need to deal with whatever symptoms or ailments cause you the most annoyance. No matter how cranky your body gets, you should make a concerted effort to learn everything there is to know about your problem and deal with it head-on. Become your own best advocate, because no one will care about your aches and pains more than you and you have to make YOU a priority. Self-care isn't selfish; it's a way of showing you love yourself.

CHAPTER 11

MOVE YOUR ASS

When you wake up and you're in pain, the last thing you want to do is get up and do practically anything. I get it. I experience it every day and I know how much the mornings can suck. But I am sorry to say that no matter how miserable you feel, you need to move. It's as important as the air you breathe.

There are days when walking in slow motion on the treadmill is all I can do. After ten minutes or so, however, I almost always feel better. I have Spotify on my phone, which allows me to listen to music from high school, and that kind of music makes me happy. I listen to The Who, Bruce Springsteen, Supertramp, KC and the Sunshine Band, Meatloaf…you never know. It depends on my mood. Recently I discovered Pit Bull, and I find his music motivating. I always make sure that my earbuds and phone are charged because listening to music makes it possible for me to get a workout in. Without music, I listen to my breathing and my whining. None of those things are helpful.

I'm pretty obsessed with the elliptical. It doesn't generally hurt my parts too badly. I get on there and can go for up to an hour. I remember my girlfriend telling me that the elliptical makes her ass and thighs huge. I could care less. I'm burning calories, getting my heartbeat stimulated, and lessening the ache that permeates in my legs. It is truly my morning savior. And I can handle my ass being a little bigger. Hell, the Kardashians have proven that big asses are in!

And thank goodness, because I have a decent-sized one for a white girl.

When your body parts are cranky, swimming is another awesome alternative. But, for me, certain requirements are necessary in order for me to go swimming. If a pool isn't at least eighty-four degrees, I can't do it. I have arthritis now, and anything cooler intensifies my body aches. I also struggle with arm and leg pain, so there are times when it helps to have a boogie board to hang on to. I never know what is going to hurt, so I need to be open-minded about my aches and pains so I can make whatever adjustments are necessary to make exercise possible.

I also love to rollerblade, but I have to be careful. If I fall, I'm screwed. Even with wrist guards and knee pads, my body doesn't appreciate falling on it anymore. One fall puts me out of commission for at least a week. I love to rollerblade along the canal path on the Genesee River in Rochester, but the city does a lousy job keeping the path clear of debris, so I have to be even more careful. In fact, I didn't rollerblade in New York at all the past two years because the path wasn't clear enough, and I was too afraid that I'd fall and get hurt.

When I rollerblade in Florida, it's usually safer for me, and my risk of falling is much less. I may be fighting high winds, but I don't usually deal with hills or debris, and rollerblading there feels safer. It's frustrating when you have a sport you love participating in, and you have to think twice because your body is so much older than your brain. And, believe me, there is a huge discrepancy between my biological age and the age in my mind.

A few years back I took a dance class. I've loved dancing ever since I was in high school, and it felt good to be back in the studio. Unfortunately, I developed a severe case of plantar fasciitis in my feet during this time, and it took close to a year for my feet to heal. It was an inconvenient injury, to say the least. I was supposed to be at my brother-in-law's wedding that summer, but I couldn't put the heels on because my feet hurt so badly. Before the wedding, I got shots of cortisone in both heels to help me be more comfortable in the shoes. Sadly, it did absolutely nothing.

It was the second time I had a cortisone shot, and I decided that cortisone sucked and didn't work on me. But I seem to be a perpetual glutton for punishment. Recently, I tried a similar injection in my neck. It was a pretty unnerving procedure that really stressed me out. When your pain is so chronic that it's virtually impossible to ignore, however, you'll try just about anything. Once again, it did nothing. Some people get a decent amount of relief with steroid injections in the neck, but it doesn't touch the pain. I had to try it, though, because I had to know whether or not it would give me some relief. It's really hard for me to be complacent about anything in my life, which is why I am constantly reading and trying new things. I feel if there is something out there that can help, I need to know.

Recently I was flying home from seeing my son and was sitting next to a retired attorney. He asked me what I did for a living, and I told him that my husband and I owned beauty salons in Rochester. When he asked me for a business card to give to his sister who lives in Rochester, the only card I had on me was the one that had the logo on it from my first book, *The Happy Hoo-Ha*. My contact information was on the back, so I gave him the card. When he saw the logo and name of the book, he burst out laughing. It is pretty funny and almost always makes people laugh or at least smile, and that makes me very happy.

I told him about The Happy Hoo-Ha trilogy and A Promise of Passion series that I had recently completed. When he asked me what I was working on now, I told him I was writing a motivational memoir about fibromyalgia. He asked me for the title. When I told him "F' You Fibro," he started laughing even harder. "It's no coincidence we were seated next to one another," he said. Apparently, he was a consultant for a company called Vital Motion that invented a device for fibromyalgia and chronic fatigue sufferers called the Hummingbird.

As it turned out, there was a huge storm in Rochester, and we were re-routed to Pittsburgh. When we landed in Pittsburgh, the airline offered us a ride back to Charlotte or told us to find our own way home. That is when I hopped in a Jeep with the attorney, his girl, and another man and drove home. In lieu of payment for the ride, I agreed to try the Hummingbird. I read all about the company and the device and agreed that it was worth trying.

The device sits under your feet and sends currents through your body. For inactive people, I think the device could be very beneficial. For me, it wasn't very helpful, but I am also one of the most active fibromyalgia sufferers you will ever meet. Some of the reviews have been very promising, and if you are a fairly sedentary person, I suggest you try it. They offer a money-back guarantee, so you really have nothing to lose.

I want to live a pain-free life, but that doesn't seem to be a scenario that I may ever experience during my lifetime because I have so many injuries. The best I can do is keep moving so that the pain I experience is more manageable. Staying active has been vital to reaching that goal. The type and amount of movement that is beneficial will be different for everyone. I just know that increased circulation brings relief. Maybe not one hundred percent relief, and the benefits from one exercise session don't last forever, but that is why you need to incorporate some type of movement into your life every single day. I have learned that I need to move my body, or it feels like the flu is freezing it into a statue of immense pain, and I don't want to live like that.

Hot yoga has been my saving grace for the past few years. I often have to modify, depending on what body part is swearing at me on any given day, but that's okay. Yoga is such a non-judgmental kind of exercise, and the community is so welcoming. The increased circulation in a warm environment is one of the most therapeutic exercises for my body. I cannot do yoga if the room isn't heated because my body becomes very stiff when it's cold, and I feel like I'm more susceptible to injury that way. Yoga increases circulation to the whole body, which can be so incredibly healing. There is yoga online, on the TV, as well as at most workout facilities these days. There are also yoga studios everywhere. You have no excuse not to at least try it.

I often try other cardio machines at the gym, but I have to be careful. I love to use the rowing machine, but when my forearms are swollen from work, the rowing machine aggravates them. I have different issues with each machine, so I have to go with what works on any given day. You cannot be rigid when it comes to working out, because your body may not always cooperate. It has a mind of its own, and you need to be resilient enough to follow your body's needs. If you accept your fluctuating limitations, you'll have better success at the gym. You also need to mix it up, so you work on different parts of your body to keep all of you healthier.

When I try new exercises, I have to be extremely cautious. My risk of injury is greater than normal people. I don't know why we are so fragile, but we are. If you accept your limitations, you can work hard and be diligent about trying to overcome them. You are stronger than you think.

CHAPTER 12

LEARNING GRATITUDE FROM SUZY

My mother is currently a ninety-three-year-old woman who travels fifty miles one way to work a few times a week. As I mentioned earlier, she has a boyfriend who is twenty-seven years her junior, owns two adorable dogs, and drives a hot sports car. She has the vibrancy and attitude of someone less than half her age. Although she has suffered many painful losses in her life, she has always focused on what she *has* and not what she *has lost*. I have to thank her for my positive attitude, because she has set such an incredible example, not only to me, but also to all of my family.

One of the things that set her apart from most older people is that she takes zero medications. She has some aches and pains (which is to be expected at her age), but, for the most part, she is healthier than most. For the past few years, however, she has had a difficult time sleeping. As of late, it has become a bigger concern for her, because, frankly, she gets pretty tired.

She recently went to a counselor to talk about her sleep issues. I don't know what you think about this, but I think it's pretty damn impressive that someone her age was open to trying something new like counseling (and potentially hypnotherapy). She met with the man one time for an hour and a half. He listened to the condensed story of her life, including all the good and bad things she had experienced.

Ironically, while she was at this appointment, I was recovering from surgery and lying in bed reading a book called *You Are a Badass* by Jen Sincero. In the book, I read a passage that I found to be very profound.

"If you are depressed, you are living in the past. If you are anxious, you are living in the future. If you are at peace, you are living in the present."

I tend to be anxious, because I do worry about tomorrow. I worry about my health, my businesses, my children, my employees, my taxes…and the list goes on. I am not a depressed person. Maybe it is because I don't lament over things that have happened in the past. After all, I know there is nothing I can do to change them. It's the whole living in the present that I try to focus on since I truly believe every day is a gift.

During my mother's session, the doctor said that he believed the key to her good health was her unrelenting gratitude. She was devastated when my dad was electrocuted, but she has never focused on the "what ifs." Like, what if she had stayed by the boat and noticed that the mast was getting too close to power lines? The what-if thing cannot change the outcome and will only drive her crazy, so she doesn't give in to it.

The doctor did believe that her worry and fear about her children's health, most particularly about my sister with terminal cancer, was the reason she was having a hard time sleeping at night. His prescription was exactly what she needed to hear. He told her to continue her ability to be grateful for today and stop worrying about tomorrow. She can't control if my sister's cancer wins. No one can. She needs to be thankful for the time she has today with her.

So, this conversation is going on as I'm reading the passage from the book. The universe is pretty crazy sometimes.

CHAPTER 13

RANDOM BITS and PIECES

When I counsel my salon clients about fibromyalgia, I always seem to have random bits of advice that I've learned over the years that have helped me cope better with this nagging ailment. As I mentioned earlier, I have a strong aversion to bright lights. I do have hazel eyes, and they say that light-eyed people can be more sensitive to light. I just know that my sensitivity is far beyond the normal person's response to brightness. It can be annoying if you're unprepared, so taking the motto of the boy scouts is not a bad idea.

There is no way I can walk onto a beach without sunglasses on. I can't physically open my eyes if there is sunshine, ocean, and some sand. The light and reflection from the water can make it literally impossible for me to open my eyes. The solution? Be prepared and always have sunglasses with you. If you keep a pair in your car or your purse, you'll always be able to protect yourself against unexpected brightness.

I have a fairly new client, whom I briefly mentioned earlier in this book, who is in her late thirties and was recently diagnosed with fibro. It was interesting how I found out how she had the condition. As I was giving her a wax, she complained that the fluorescent lights on my ceiling were bugging her eyes. I admit they are bright, which I like because it helps me find stray hairs that I miss. And since I don't look directly up at them, they've never bothered me before. I could totally sympathize with her. She said that her aversion to light was new, and it was really a nuisance. Yep, it sure can be. The solution? She now wears sunglasses during her waxes, and the uncomfortable sensation in her eyes isn't an issue. She may feel some discomfort during her Brazilian wax because it is a service that removes her pubic hair from the root, but that is to be expected. I totally understood her legitimate visual discomfort and completely sympathized with her situation.

Do you like how I refer to pain as discomfort? In my opinion, if you keep referring to all the pain you are experiencing as this hellacious devil who is lighting fires of misery in your limbs, then you are reinforcing negativity and focusing on all the bad things going on, which will only make you feel shittier. For example, I often experience a burning sensation in my upper back, neck, and shoulders when I blow-dry my hair. I usually have to get in strange positions to use the round brush to style my hair properly because the pain can be so intense. It's a hard sensation to accurately describe. Suffice it to say, it feels like acid is traveling in my bloodstream, and it can be debilitating at times. When I am in a lot of pain and know that I can't keep my arms up, I will let my hair dry naturally and then use a large-barreled curling iron to complete my hairstyle. This way I can section my hair and curl it in parts while taking breaks in between so I can finish the style. It often works better that way because I can curl part of it, rest, do something else for a minute, and then go back to it. If you budget your time, you'll be able to work it into your morning routine without letting it cause you frustration or make you late to work. Once my hair is finished, I always feel prettier. If I just said fuck it and didn't style my hair before work, I would feel lousier every time I looked in the mirror throughout the day. And, believe me, there are mirrors EVERYWHERE in our beauty salons, so I am seeing my reflection from every direction—and sometimes it feels daunting.

I want to make it clear that I don't blame fibro for my pain when I'm doing my hair. On the contrary, I blame the neck injury that happened in 2008 when I was waxing that woman's v-j-jay…

There is also a benefit to marrying a hairdresser. Lately, my husband has been finishing my hair in the mornings because he recognizes how uncomfortable I am trying to hold my arms above my head. Even if your significant other is not a hairdresser, you could always employ them to help you out with this task. For some people, it may even be fun. Think of it as another way to bond, and maybe let it become part of foreplay. Rewarding your significant for their efforts is a great idea. And I can say this from first-hand experience.

Human touch is extremely important and I'm sorry if you, the reader, are a single person who doesn't get to experience the touch or attention of another person. I am comfortable being alone, but I also treasure the moments when I am being caressed and loved. But if you are alone, I'd suggest you get a pet. There is something very therapeutic about interacting with a furry animal. That is one of the reasons they bring therapy dogs to hospitals and nursing homes. Being able to hold and pet an animal can be healing. I've had dogs, cats, and even guinea pigs that have brought a tremendous amount of joy and comfort to my life. It can be very relaxing and enjoyable to cuddle with an animal, so maybe it is something to consider. Furthermore, you can't put a price on the unconditional love of an animal.

I'm fortunate to be in a very affectionate relationship, so I get a lot of loving touch throughout my day. When my husband and I are in bed having coffee in the morning, he usually reaches over and rubs my neck, which is always stiff when I wake up. At night, he'll often rub my hands, because they are almost always swollen at the end of the day. It's not like he gives some kind of intense massage. He simply touches the area that is grumpy, and it makes me feel so much better. The pain doesn't remarkably disappear, but there are definitely healing powers to a loving touch. If you do live alone, I recommend that you get a therapeutic massage once in a while, because it can be very restorative. Not only is the touch of a massage therapist's hands important, but so also are the healing powers of getting your circulation stimulated. You can't heal if you are sedentary and your body is stagnant.

Both of my sons currently have large dogs, like sixty to seventy pounds apiece, and I can't believe how awesome it is to cuddle with a big dog. I've always owned little pups, like Maltese, which is more like hugging a little baby. When you curl up next to a seventy-pound dog that thinks he is a baby, however, it feels like you're hugging a person. I am so hooked on this big dog thing now that I completely understand the appeal.

I need to reiterate how important it is to be forgiving of yourself and your not-so-perfect body. If you are performing a task that is taxing on your body, you may be forced to cease what you're doing, and that is okay. You need to give yourself permission to listen to what your body is telling you. For example, I have finally realized that most of the time when I vacuum, my upper body hurts (it's that acid sensation I was talking about). Vacuuming is one household chore that I really dislike because it causes me quite a bit of discomfort. Sometimes it isn't too uncomfortable, but other times I just have to stop. And believe me, I've spent good money on all different types of vacuums to make my life easier. To make matters worse, since I have a large house, by the time I finish vacuuming, my upper body may ache for hours afterwards. It's just not worth it. So, I made the choice to either have someone else do it or wait to do it until a day that I feel better and confident that it won't piss off my limbs. Sometimes you have to give yourself a break. What's more important? Your sense of well-being or a few cookie crumbs on the floor? Okay, I don't eat cookies, but you know what I mean.

Don't be embarrassed to ask for help. There are certain things that you will find are nearly impossible to do. For example, I pretty much cannot open any jar unless I can smash it on the countertop first to loosen the seal and then say a little prayer that the jar doesn't break (I have broken a few in my lifetime). Even then I can't always open it. Pickle jars have been a nemesis for years. If you live alone, invite a friend over and ask them to loosen up any of the jars or containers that are giving you a difficult time. They even make special jar openers designed for people with arthritis or other hand-related disabilities. I wasn't a huge fan of the apparatus because jars come in so many different widths, but I'm sure they have improved the design since I last bought one. For now, I smash jars on the counter or the floor or I bug my husband or kids to open things for me.

If there is a childproof top on your medication (which means that only a child has enough finesse or strength to open the damn bottle), just leave the lid slightly ajar so it's easier to open the next time. As long as you don't tip the meds over, and they fall on the floor, there really isn't a need to screw on a cap back to its original position unless it specifically says to seal securely for potency's sake.

I've been completely annoyed with the new bra styles at Victoria's Secret because they have this fancy "V"-type clasp in the front. I have three problems with this "clever" new design which pisses me off every time I wear a front-closure bra. One, I can never find where to put the parts together unless I have my glasses on (and I still have to squint), because the dang hole is too small to see. Secondly, it hurts my hands to try to hold it close enough to even match up the two parts. Thirdly, even once I find the hole, I have issues getting the two parts to go together properly. I can't tell you how many times I've asked my husband to help me put my bra on because, apparently, I'm severely challenged when it comes to dressing myself. To me, the secret behind Victoria's bras is that there must be a secret to getting the damn thing that no one has shared with yours truly yet.

Speaking of dressing myself, zippers around the back of my body are another source of frustration. Between my neck injury and a little tendonitis in my shoulders, reaching behind my back is nearly impossible. If Mark isn't around to zip me up, I will go to work unzipped and have one of my staff members do it for me. I try to maintain my flexibility, but reaching behind the upper part of my back is difficult for me.

Have any of you ever had issues getting your toothpaste out? Sometimes I feel like a very old woman when it comes to some of the more trivial tasks that I perform daily. It hurts my hands to squeeze out the toothpaste, so I have gotten in the habit of rolling it up from the end.

Mind you, there are times when I am too vigorous with my rolling technique, and I have enough toothpaste squirting out of the end to brush a crocodile's set of choppers, but it's better than squeezing from the middle and having nothing come out. It's the same with some of my facial products. Mark & M.E. (that's the name of our salon) has its own skincare line, and the exfoliating scrubs come in tubes similar to toothpaste. Since they are thick, it takes a fair amount of strength to get the product out. My solution? I keep my scrubs in the shower, and I step on them to get them out. It's the only way I have figured out how to do it. Sounds silly but it works.

After I brush my teeth, I generally put on my makeup. I have two parts of my makeup routine that are difficult. I have a really hard time opening up the containers that house the blush and the eyeshadows. I tend to leave the containers open all of the time or break the mechanism that holds the two parts together because I'm tired of struggling with the damn things. I have a friend who has found incredible success selling Mary Kay products. I hadn't tried their makeup for years, so I thought I'd give her some business and buy some things. The makeup was fine, but the packaging sucked. I had to break the containers that held both the blush and the eye shadows because I could never get the stupid things open. I told her that they needed new designs to make the makeup more user-friendly for people who have arthritic hands.

I also struggle with holding my arms up to put my mascara on. I feel the ache from my neck to my hands when I hold my arms up for too long. I love that we offer eyelash extensions at our salon because that takes one more annoying chore out of my daily routine. Finding alternatives to making your life easier and less painful should be a priority. As of late, I don't wear extensions but I'm really good at using both hands to put mascara on.

I don't mind doing laundry. I'm fortunate because our washer and dryer are in a small room attached to our bedroom. I have no problems folding laundry or putting things away either. The only laundry that I don't like to fold is my sheets. Face it, you're never going to get the sheets to be folded as neatly as they come when you buy them at the store. If you are capable of folding them that well, you need a reward. As soon as I take sheets out of the package, I marvel at how they were ever able to fit inside the plastic to begin with. I think the problem with the sheets is how big they are. There is something about expanding my arms to fold them somewhat decently that aggravates me. The better solution is to wash the sheets and put them right back on the bed, so you don't have to fold them. Sadly, it's a struggle for me to put the fitted sheet on a bed, but it's just another task that I take my time with or ask for help with.

I'm trying to share as many scenarios as possible so you can understand that your limitations don't have to stop you from living. You just need to figure out strategies that will help you stay productive, because if you stop doing things, you will die.

Stairs can be tough. If I eat something that aggravates my fibro (like beer, pasta, or cooked tomato sauce), it feels like there is poison in my legs when I walk up the stairs to go to bed at night. I have crappy, arthritic knees, but I am pretty good at ignoring that kind of knee pain when I walk up or down the stairs. It's the ache that bothers me the most. I definitely need to consider a ranch if I get myself another home for those illustrious golden years because I know that climbing stairs on a daily basis could be a problem. A few years ago, my husband and I were considering buying a second home in Florida. I found a gorgeous two-story home on the water in the Sarasota area. When he saw the pictures of this house, he agreed it was a beautiful home, but said we HAD to buy a ranch, or he would be forced to carry me up and down the stairs. Even if I don't want to admit it, he is right. Chances are, stairs will become even more difficult as time passes, especially since I'm already having difficulties. I hate thinking that way, but I need to be realistic. I may have a twenty-five-year-old brain, but I sure as hell don't have a twenty-five-year-old body.

As a resident of upstate New York, I have the distinct pleasure of dealing with snow in the wintertime. I'm not a huge fan of the cold, but I love Rochester, so I suck it up and take as many vacations to warm weather as possible. Fortunately, my husband takes care of all the shoveling. If he weren't around, I'd have to find someone to do it. It's a job that hurts my upper body, and frankly, I hate the cold weather and can't stand to shovel.

I'm grateful that I can read on my iPhone because I have a tough time holding a book open. Since I read on a daily basis, this was a huge adjustment for me. I used an iPad for a while, but even that was too large for me to hold without hurting my hands. If I do read a paperback book, I've gotten used to breaking the binding so I can hold it open. That seems wrong to me, however, so I've shied away from reading physical books. I stick to the remarkable little rectangle because it doesn't aggravate my hands as profoundly—especially since I read every day and refuse to give it up.

When I had an hour's break at the salon the other day, I decided to work on this book. I was really uncomfortable in the chair because it was the wrong height, and my hips were achy. I got a small pillow and put it under my seat, and I felt a lot better. It amazes me that I ever need a pillow because I have a fair amount of junk in my trunk, but those hips need some extra cushion sometimes. I also find myself using small pillows behind my low back for extra lumbar support. If you aren't comfortable, don't be complacent—find some kind of prop that you can use that will make you feel better. Don't be reactive and pissed off, be proactive and figure out something that makes you feel better.

Sometimes I laugh when I physically can't squeeze the juice out of a lemon, but have no problem waxing the Afro off a 350-pound woman's bikini line. I guess since I get paid to do Brazilians, then I have extra incentive to be able to finish each client safely and efficiently, and no one actually pays me to squeeze lemons. But I like to cook, and I don't like bottled lemon juice, so I had to figure it out. I bought an electric lemon juicer to make my life easier, since I use a lot of fresh lemon juice in my cooking. It's a pretty cool kitchen aid, although I hate cleaning it.

When I don't feel like squeezing lemons (or limes for that matter), I'm fortunate to live next to a Wegmans Supermarket, and they do it for me.

Another thing that has offered me some relief is Epsom salt baths. People have used Epsom salts for hundreds of years to help with aches and pains. When the salts are added to water, it breaks down into magnesium and sulfate. These compounds permeate into your skin, and, for me, help to alleviate some of my nightly aches and pains. I have jets attached to my tub to circulate the water, but it works in a regular tub as well. Anything that can get our circulation going is beneficial. It's also a good idea to stretch while you're soaking in the water, or right after, while your muscles are relaxed and warm. If you aren't a fan of baths, that's okay. You can always do an Epsom salt wrap on your body. Get a towel wet with hot water, put some salts on the towel, and wrap your knee, hands, neck, etc. with the towel, and you should find some relief.

If you're willing to put in a little effort, you'd be surprised how much relief you can get.

I may not have a PhD in wellness or health, but I'm an educated woman who takes her health very seriously. In this chapter, I've rambled on about some of the changes I've made in my life that have made me feel better, and my intent is not to have you mimic me because we all have unique bodies, and what works for me may not work for you. I hope that if even one suggestion helps you feel a little better or gives you an AHA moment, then I have done the job I set out to do. Even a *little* better is better than no change at all. I am hoping to offer you tools to make your life better, no matter how minor or slight the change may be.

Years ago, I started making sure I had water in two places—next to my bed and in my car. I have found that the more hydrated my body is, the better I feel. And isn't that what we are searching for? Feeling better and living a more fulfilling life is a goal each and every one of us should be striving towards. And I find that I really do like to drink and drive—when it's water that I'm drinking. When I was in beauty school, they said I shouldn't drink out of a straw because it could cause more wrinkles around my mouth. However, I found that I drink more when I use straws, so screw it. The benefits of staying hydrated far outweigh any concerns I have. I even have a few straws in my briefcase so I'm never without. Whatever gets you to stay hydrated, do it.

Another random thing that I don't do is chew gum. It hurts my jaw, and I have made the conscious decision that if a given action causes something to hurt, then I try to avoid it. I also hate the way people look when they chew gum, so I don't feel bad not participating in the habit.

One day, a woman walked into the salon, and her phone rang. She excused herself because it was a call she had been waiting on for a few hours. Ironically, it was a rheumatology office scheduling an appointment. Apparently, the woman was just diagnosed with fibro by her primary care physician and was now being sent to a rheumatologist for a follow-up consultation. She is an attorney in her late thirties, who is married and has two children. We had a very long talk about the implications of living with fibro and some of the coping mechanisms I use to be able to be a productive woman who doesn't succumb to this bizarre affliction. I also shared some of the triggers that cause flare-ups in my life. I couldn't emphasize enough how important it was for her to recognize what stressors triggered the change in her body. I understand that it's virtually impossible to completely eliminate stress from your life, but it's vital that you diligently and consciously try to have some control over the issues that cause you stress, so you have a chance of managing your pain. Take those imaginary earbuds out of your ears and really try to listen to what your body is trying to tell you. I think we, as women especially, tend to be very hard on ourselves. We are wives, mothers, workers, housekeepers, taxicab drivers, and the list goes on. When you're feeling like shit, honor that feeling and be forgiving. You don't have to be a superwoman every day, no matter how much you want to be. There will be days when you don't feel like doing anything physical, but that doesn't mean you can't play cards or watch a movie. Please try to be open-minded to change, and don't get caught up in such a rigid life that you can't be flexible when your body isn't cooperating. Some days you will feel normal, and other days, you're going to feel like shit.

Since she was newly diagnosed, she was having difficulties emotionally and psychologically wrapping her head around her new health condition, in addition to the physical changes that were happening in her body. The initial diagnosis is difficult to process, especially since it is such a strange and obscure condition. She was surprised I suffered with it since I seemed so upbeat and okay. I assured her that I make the conscientious decision every single day to not let it stop me from doing what I want to do. I may have limitations, but I focus on being positive. I felt like a cheerleader offering her hope and encouragement, but that is my purpose when I meet anyone who is dealing with this diagnosis or a similar ailment. Even if your body isn't cooperating, you and you alone can control whether you have a good or bad attitude. I choose a good one.

It's funny because I think about the elderly quite often when I struggle with everyday tasks. Like changing the toilet paper, for instance. The spring mechanism bothers my hand. The problem is that I'm the type of person who gets thoroughly annoyed when someone finishes the roll and doesn't put a new one on. There is something about an empty roll that drives me crazy. But at night (and sometimes during the day) when my hands are swollen, I'll steal some paper from a new roll, so I don't finish off the one that is almost empty. I let the next person change it for me. It's better than leaving it empty, right?

I really love to write, but I worry that one day I won't be able to continue writing books without a lot of pain. Although I enjoy the act of using my fingers to put words down, I know there may be a time when I will have to employ some kind of voice-activated system on my computer. I don't want to ever stop writing, but there is a possibility that my hands won't be cooperative.

As of right now, I am typing away on my laptop and loving it. Writing makes me happy, so I keep doing it. And if someone reads something I've written and enjoys it, all the better.

Fibro sufferers often have aversions to smells. As I said earlier, I haven't worn cologne in years because I cannot tolerate any strong smells on me. Back in the day, I used to wear my husband's cologne because I could never find a woman's scent that I liked. Several years ago, however, I stopped wearing any type of fragrance altogether because they would cause an instant headache and nausea. I also refrain from fragrant body lotions. They have the same effect on me. Artificial smells make me feel sick. It's funny because so many people get into routines, like putting perfume on every day, that it is difficult to break the habit. But if the habit is causing you discomfort…

We often have issues with textures as well. I need things to be soft. You will never catch this woman in any type of wool clothing. Even the thought of it makes me feel scratchy and uncomfortable. Lace bras are also a source of frustration. No matter how sexy a lace bra may be, my need to take it off completely negates any sexiness that comes with wearing one. I'm also weird about the softness of my pillow. I can't handle anything too hard. I like overly soft blankets and comforters. Basically, I like warm, cozy textures that are soft and gentle. Anything rough or hard is best left on the barn floor.

Loud noises can be another source of aggravation. Sometimes listening to kids yelling can make me a little crazy. I had a young woman come in for a Brazilian recently who was screaming like she was being murdered. To make matters worse, she would sit up and scream in my face after each strip was removed. After the fourth rip, I told her that she was only getting a bikini and I left the room. I couldn't take it. She was uncooperative and annoying as hell, and it wasn't worth it for me to try to finish the service. That hasn't happened very often in my career, but sometimes you have to make those kinds of uncomfortable decisions.

My mother was always a huge fan of us using our library voices. She never liked anyone to raise his or her voice in or out of the house. Well, I guess I'm becoming more like my mother every day. And that is okay with me. My mom (also known as Grandma Suzy) is the coolest ninety-three-year-old you would ever have the pleasure of meeting, and I'd never criticize her for having a sensitivity to loud noises. Living in a no-judgment zone is the best way to live. You never know what someone else is going through as much as you will never understand what I have gone through in my life. I try very hard not to judge others, because I hate being judged.

Besides, love is so much better than hate.

CHAPTER 14

IT'S IN YOUR HEAD

Istruggled for a lot of years with the notion that maybe all my ailments were psychosomatic. It never really made sense that any woman who wasn't in a major accident or who wasn't born with a debilitating condition should be this messed up. I have to give a huge shout-out to the family I was born into for not thinking I was crazy. I'm also fortunate that the husband I married always believed me and didn't think it was necessary to commit me to the R wing, although I'm quite certain he considered it sometimes. I totally get the skeptics out there. We look fine. We act fine. I really do get it. But our struggle is real, no matter what we may look like on the outside or how we act. The biggest thing between me and others who suffer from this condition is that I see myself as a survivor, I feel blessed I don't have a terminal disease, I want to enjoy life in spite of my limitations, and I will NEVER give up fighting to live my best life. I choose happiness, and I want you too also.

I've always believed that there was something inherently weaker in some part of my body that has led to this affliction. When I hear that places like the Mayo Clinic are doing research on fibromyalgia, I get pretty giddy. Our predicament has been legitimized once and for all. It took a long time for that to happen. Now that I hear there are plausible explanations of why this is happening to us, I can barely contain my joy.

One of my clients with fibro was evaluated at the Mayo Clinic recently and the doctors told her that the neurons in the thalamus of fibro patients are over-stimulated. And since the thalamus relays our body's sensory information, such as sound, touch, sight, etc. This is why we perceive pain so readily and are so sensitive to external and internal stimuli. (Please forgive me if my interpretation is not exact. I'm not a doctor, and this is how I processed this explanation). This is the first time in decades that I wholeheartedly believe in someone's assessment of why this happens to us. The part of the brain that interprets touch, pain, and temperature is continually amped up, and that is why we are more sensitive. We are always in fight or flight mode, which is an extremely accurate description of how I operate daily. I feel a lingering sense of panic, even in bed at night. Their explanation makes so much sense and I was thrilled to blame it on my brain. Who would have thought that my thalamus was responsible for making me uber-sensitive to just about everything? It makes total sense. Even if there isn't a definitive cure, it is so reassuring to know that I'm not alone and I'm not crazy.

Now we need to figure out how to get our thalamus to calm the fuck down so we can be productive and happy members of society. The doctors instructed my client to do calming exercises like yoga and meditation. As I mentioned earlier, I haven't mastered the meditation thing yet, but yoga on a regular basis is very healing. Yoga also helps with my circulation issues in a much healthier way than Gabapentin. I've tried that medication a few times, and it wasn't my friend. It didn't help and the side effects were not worth it.

The research is not conclusive, but I've read articles that say anywhere between four and eleven million people suffer from fibromyalgia, and most are women. That is a staggering number of people, regardless of what number is more accurate. Honestly, I wouldn't be surprised if there were even more of us around. There are so many stressors in our lives, personally, locally, and globally, that there are times when it is impossible NOT to feel some form of anxiety. What I am most pleased about is that our situation has been recognized and I'm ecstatic that legitimate research is being conducted to help us find some relief.

CHAPTER 15

MEDICAL MARIJUANA

One of my husband's clients has suffered from a hip condition her entire life. As she entered her thirties, the pain became unbearable. She was introduced to a local healthcare provider who was able to provide her with a medical marijuana card. As she was explaining how much better she was feeling and how much better she was sleeping, Mark made a point of having us talk. She gave me the woman's name, and I called her right away.

For some reason, it felt really awkward making an appointment to get one of these cards. I can't explain why. Although I definitely have some legitimate ailments going on, the whole idea of asking for marijuana from a doctor seemed odd and slightly uncomfortable. When I called the office, she asked me what was wrong with me that would warrant my need for the card. I told her I had fibro, osteoarthritis, tendonitis, and tenosynovitis, and then I laughed and told her I had all of the "itises." Once my list of ailments was recorded, she told me that I needed my doctor to send over proof that I have been seen for some of these issues. Furthermore, I was to have the office send over a list of all the medications I was on. When I told her that I didn't take any medications, she reiterated how imperative it was to include all of my prescriptions with my information. Once again, I told her I didn't take any kind of prescription medications. Her response was, "Even with all that is wrong with you?" Yep, even with all that is wrong with me. I'm a freak, I get it.

Our family doctor never seemed supportive of regular marijuana when it came up in discussions with my kids, so I wasn't sure how he'd feel about me wanting to use a medical-grade alternative. When I called the secretary, who has worked with him for years, I told her I needed a favor. She has always been extremely pleasant and accommodating so I was confident she'd help me out. I whispered into the phone when I was speaking with her, which seems ridiculous since I'm in my fifties and shouldn't be embarrassed by my request. I think I wanted to make sure my doctor didn't overhear that I was trying to get a medical marijuana card. I told her that I needed proof that I was fucked up (yep, those were my exact words). She burst out laughing before she asked what "kind of proof" I needed to share with them. Basically, they wanted information about my last two visits that would substantiate my claim that I indeed had medical problems that could be improved by the use of medical marijuana. She pulled up my chart and said there was a pretty long list of problems. The way she said it was kind of funny, so I asked her what kinds of things were listed. The first thing on the list was spondylitis. That was one that threw me for a loop. She stopped and remarked that she wasn't even sure what that was. Her admission made me laugh because I wasn't positive which ailment that referred to either. I suspected it had to do with my degenerated back, but I wasn't exactly sure and knew I would have to look that one up. She continued to read the list and we collectively agreed that I had enough problems that would warrant the card. Yes, we had substantiated proof that I was legitimately fucked up.

It took a few months to get an appointment, which proved how popular the use of medical marijuana has become. Getting legal pot was a lot more in demand than I thought, but I think that's a good thing, since I'm pretty anti-meds. The morning of the appointment, I felt anxious. I was hoping this would be the answer I was looking for and I knew I'd be extremely disappointed if it didn't help. Smoking home-grown pot hadn't worked well for me over the past couple of years, so I really prayed that this alternative would provide me with some relief.

There are actually two reasons why smoking pot hasn't always been the answer for me. The first problem with any kind of inhalation is my lungs. After smoking like a chimney in high school and then inhaling acrylic nail products for over twenty years, my lungs aren't great. Smoking anything elicits deep, masculine-sounding coughs that make it sound like I've been inhaling Cuban cigars for my entire life. When the effects first kick in, however, I feel relaxed and can often fall asleep. It also has been very helpful with my libido, which is always a positive side effect that I'll never complain about. My problem is that after the high wears off, I often feel worse than before I smoked it. The dehydration reaction that I sometimes experience is brutal. In addition, I often get violently achy like I've been plagued by the flu. On top of that, sometimes I experience weakness in my limbs. Once again, it's that flu-like sensation that so many of us experience and try to avoid. What I have learned since starting this book is that I need to drink more water if I smoke, and I can't succumb to salty munchies that can lead to more dehydration.

The physician I met with was very nice. She asked me to list all the different types of things I have tried to help with my pain. I listed the myriads of treatments, medications, herbs, chelation, chiropractic, massage, acupuncture, elimination diets, and the list goes on and on… She was impressed by how knowledgeable I was about health, nutrition, and both Western and Eastern medicine. She told me about a medical marijuana study that was done in Europe. There wasn't a large population tested, but the results were interesting. All of the people in the study had fibromyalgia. After a consistent ritual of using medical marijuana, fifty percent said they felt one hundred percent better, and the other half said they felt fifty percent better. Damn, I'd take fifty percent any day of the week. I was even more ready to try this route.

There were two dispensaries in Rochester at this time, and once I filled out the forms online, I was good to go. Now I had to figure out what I was going to try and what I could expect from using the products.

I didn't know what to expect when I went to the facility. It was located at the back of a large brick building which I had never been to before. I had to walk through a rundown, narrow alley to find the location. There were no people walking around nor many cars parked in the parking area at the front of the lot. To be honest, the whole thing felt very sketchy. The location and look of the building added to my anxiety about going into this unknown environment and purchasing medical marijuana. I wished I had brought my husband with me. When I entered, the gentleman who greeted me was very soft-spoken and pleasant, and I instantly felt more at ease. He took my information, and I was guided to a semi-private area to talk to a pharmacist. We discussed the variety of products they offered, which were dependent on my ailments and my needs. It was overwhelming, to say the least. I couldn't believe all of the different products that were available to me. There were products geared to help me with the pain during the day and there were also products designed to help me sleep. For the nighttime, I got pills and lozenges, and for the daytime, I got a vaporizer "pen" and a vial of liquid tincture. It was expensive, but I didn't care. It was pretty exciting to think that I might actually sleep for more than a couple of hours in a row!

As soon as I got home, I tried out the pen. Needless to say, one hit and I was choking my brains out. I was only supposed to inhale lightly for three seconds, but I inhaled more like I was sucking on a four-foot bong, and that was a big mistake. There was no need to suck as hard as I did, but I didn't know how the pen worked. I know now, that's for sure. She said it usually took about fifteen minutes to kick in. She wasn't kidding. After one long inhalation and several minutes of trying to cough up a lung, I felt high. It was a nice, calm feeling, but I knew right away that this was not something I could use during the day. I have a busy life and there was no time during my day to have a foggy brain. Besides, the burning in my chest was not something I wanted to experience on a regular basis.

It's funny because I remember that day like it was yesterday. It was a Saturday after work when I brought my merchandise home. I sat at my desk to do my usual end-of-the-day bookwork, and after my single inhalation kicked in, there was no way I was tallying up the weekly sales and the staff's pay. It was pretty comical actually. Our normal routine on Saturdays is for me to do one to two hours of bookwork after work and then we go out to dinner. It was obvious that our routine was going to be quite a bit different this day. I experienced a far too relaxed brain to concentrate and a fairly aggressive sense of the munchies. I knew the bookwork would have to wait until morning, and since I was hungry, we went to an early dinner.

Normally, I drive whenever my husband and I are in a car together because I'm not a fan of the way he drives. On this day, there was no way I was going to get behind the wheel. Yep, all from one exaggerated toke. We sat at the bar and got a drink. I was feeling good. Especially after I curbed my munchies with some food.

Now that I realized the pen probably wasn't the answer, I tried the tincture. That was one of the grossest things I have ever put under my tongue. For those of you who have smoked pot before, imagine what used bong water would taste like if it was thickened with an additive that resembled decaying sewage, and then you voluntarily ingested it. For those of you who have never smoked pot before, imagine putting a few drops of thick, pungent swamp water under your tongue. It was so foul that I couldn't brush my teeth, tongue, and gums thoroughly enough. I knew this probably wouldn't be the answer either. And, to top it off, this tiny (and I mean TINY) bottle cost ninety dollars. No thanks.

Although the daytime regimes were a bust, I had two more options for nighttime relief that I was hoping would help. The first night I took one of the capsules. It had a 20–1 ratio of CBD to THC. She told me it would take about forty-five minutes to kick in, and that was exactly how long it took. That night I slept for four hours straight, which isn't common in my world, and felt pretty damn good. I continued to take it every night, but I still wasn't getting enough uninterrupted sleep. My next option was the lozenges. They were honey flavored, and are supposed to take about the same amount of time to kick in. They affected me much more strongly and I fell asleep with a lot less restlessness.

Even though I continued with the regimen of one or the other, I was still incapable of sleeping more than three or four hours at a time. I had to ask myself if my body would simply take longer to adjust to longer sleep patterns, since it wasn't used to any prolonged amount of sleep. Since I suffered from erratic sleep for most of my life, it made sense that it might take longer for me to learn how to sleep through the night like a normal person. Although the pharmacist told me that the nighttime products should last eight hours, that was not what I experienced. For me, four hours was the max.

I went back to the dispensary to buy some more supplies and to talk to them about alternative approaches to find more success with the products. At first, the pharmacist suggested I take a hit off of the pen when I woke up the first time and maybe that would help me. I told her that I had lung issues, so that wasn't the best idea. She suggested a second pill. When I tried that, I found it difficult to get up in the morning. I detest feeling groggy and lethargic, so a second pill at two a.m. was not the answer either.

I also think that our bodies get used to a drug when it's used on a regular basis and, after a while, it can become less effective. This is why I tried to alternate between a few different products. I also skipped taking them on nights that I've had too much alcohol because the combination can cause me to become profoundly dizzy. I never figured out the perfect concoction, but it helped for a few months. Since then, I've discontinued going to the store and have let my card expire. The products were just too damn expensive and weren't as helpful as I had hoped.

Over the next few months, I shared my experience with a multitude of other medical marijuana users. There are a lot of people who find tremendous relief from them. It could be a great alternative for you as well. I guess my body is just finicky—which is another annoying fibro trait.

As I said, this shit is expensive. I spent around three hundred dollars a month on my supplies, which I understand not everyone can do. In the months to come, I only bought the products aimed at helping me sleep better, because I really didn't like anything that impaired my ability to think clearly during the day. They are developing new products all the time with different ratios and strengths, so I didn't give up on it right away. I got my card in the fall of 2019 and probably spent close to three thousand dollars before I realized that it wasn't worth the money. Now that it is 2023, things have changed, and marijuana products are readily available to the general public. I definitely think they are worth trying out. You just need to figure out what works for you, and what doesn't.

CHAPTER 16

MY SECRET TO HAPPY

If you're feeling sorry for me in any way, shape, or form, DON'T. I wanted to share my story with you in order to give you an idea of what I've gone through in the hope that I can help you in some way—no matter how small the help may be. There are a gazillion people out there with much bigger problems than I have. I know that I listed a long list of issues that I've had to deal with, but I constantly remind myself that, as of now, none of them are life-threatening. For that, I am extremely grateful. My overabundant collection of maladies is just annoying, uncomfortable, and a big pain in the ass (actually my ass is one part of me that doesn't hurt—at least for now. My hips, on the other hand…). The secret is to find a way to deal with your symptoms with as little medication as possible, constantly fight to take care of your body through nutrition, exercise, and relaxation techniques, and to listen—and I mean REALLY listen to what your body is telling you. You have so much more power than you think, and you need to start thinking with more determination and steadfast positivity. My advice may not be rocket science, but it's real, and it works for me. Since you took the time to read this book, then you probably needed to hear some positivity and encouragement and also the reinforcement that you are NOT alone! Does something always hurt? Yep. Do I let it stop me from being happy? No fucking way.

I know that I rambled on and on about all the shit I've been through in my life, but I also know countless men and women have experienced as much or way more than what I've gone through. My goal is to give you hope, because I believe that once we lose hope, it's over, and you might as well find the tallest bridge to swan dive off of (please note that was a figurative suggestion and I pray no one ever gives up the fight). I acknowledge that you may be limited in what you can do, but that doesn't mean there aren't alternatives to help you find a little light at the end of your proverbial tunnel. Additionally, you need to remind yourself that your tunnel in life does not have to lead you into hell. Our time on this earth is too precious to give in and, more importantly, to give up.

My knees are shot, and I can't run, but that is okay. Instead, I walk on a treadmill. Sometimes I walk fast, sometimes I walk with an incline, and there are other times that I walk slowly. The most important thing is that I am moving. And never stop telling yourself that motion is lotion and movement can be magic. Since I was never a huge fan of running, I don't miss it. But just because running isn't an option doesn't mean I can't find another type of cardio exercise. Hell, if you walk fast enough, you'll get your heart rate up, and that can be a game changer.

My sister has terminal cancer, and the prognosis is bleak. It is a situation that has devastated me in ways that I can't even put into words because it is too overwhelming to talk about. The sadness I feel for her and her family is insurmountable. Cancer terrifies me. It is cruel, ugly, and unforgiving. No one should have to experience what she is going through. That is a woman to pray for—not me. But even with her horrific diagnosis, she is a fighter. She fights every day to enjoy the people that she loves and cherishes every moment on this earth. Pretty amazing, wouldn't you say?

More than anything, I want you to believe that you don't have to let fibro consume your life. Because if it does, it will win. Will it make certain activities difficult? Of course, it will. It will also cause you to make changes in your life that you may not want to. But if you aren't open-minded enough to make those changes and be willing to adapt, then you probably aren't going to get much out of my stories. I thrive on being organized and regimented, but there are times when I have to be willing to give in or make adjustments. Try to act like a Darwinian animal and force yourself to adapt to the cards you've been dealt. If I were a gambler, I would bet on YOU. Now I need you to bet on yourself as well.

I cannot say it enough that you absolutely do have more control over your body than you think, and you absolutely have even more control over your mind. Fibromyalgia doesn't have a "Stage 4" label associated with it and will not give a time frame for when your life will be over. Don't let the label that your physicians awarded to your condition define you, or it will have all of the power. If you give up the power that you inherently possess, then you are ultimately allowing it to dictate your future. Most importantly, if you allow it to monopolize your life, you won't have much of a life that is worth living. I believe that we have the innate ability to make our situation bearable and even better. I'm always striving to be the winner of my body, and I want you to do everything in your power to try to feel the same way. If you succumb to the diagnosis and hide under the covers, it wins. Please don't let it. Make yourself the winner and not some weird-ass condition that no one can pronounce, let alone spell.

Be honest with yourself when you answer the following question. Have you ever considered that it is possible to defy the odds by figuring out strategies to beat this bitch? That has been my quest for as long as I can remember, and that is another reason I am sharing my story. I truly believe I have taken this bitch down. It no longer antagonizes me regularly, and I don't let it stop me from living a productive and happy life.

Once again, let me reiterate the secrets to my success in overcoming this bizarre affliction, because, once I made conscientious changes to my diet and exercise regime as well as my mental outlook on my situation, I'm not convinced fibromyalgia is even a problem for me anymore. I have what I like to refer to as a lot of mechanical problems with my body. However, as long as I stay hydrated, avoid beer, red sauces, artificial sweeteners, and fried or processed food, all while staying active, my fibro symptoms are pretty much non-existent. It seems so simple, doesn't it? But I know it's not. If you like fast food, you have to limit your consumption because your body can't tolerate crap, and that's what fast food is. You can't lie around all day doing nothing, hoping things will change, because they never will. They will only get worse. You have to move your ass, my friends, and make sure you drink at least one hundred ounces of water every day. Not juices. Not soda. Not energy drinks (which are total poison in my opinion). Just water.

If you want a hard-ass motivational story, check out David Goggin's book *Can't Hurt Me.* I've read it twice so far and will probably read it again. Goggins is hardcore and will probably be too intense for many of you, but his message is extraordinary and potentially life-changing. I read this book as I was struggling to deal with the menopausal changes that were plaguing my body and the frustrating new issues I was dealing with. He accomplished countless physical feats in his life that seemed absolutely impossible. I found his story unbelievably compelling. He defied insurmountable odds and successfully completed tasks that most people wouldn't have had the courage to try in the first place. I cried reading most of his book. He was a poor boy from Buffalo, New York (my hometown), who was neglected and beaten badly by his own father. He was also uneducated and cheated his way through school. Ultimately, he went on to find success in spite of his absolutely horrifying indoctrination to life and a slew of physical, emotional, and psychological trauma. Not only do I applaud his perseverance and tenacity, I admire his courage.

My youngest son told me about Goggins a few years ago, and since then, I've become a huge fan. He ran one-hundred-mile races (which I cannot even fathom anyone doing) and persevered through challenging injuries that would have been crippling to most people. He proved that with hard work and a determined mindset, you have so much more ability and so much more strength than you could ever imagine. He overcame incredibly horrific obstacles, and I am a true believer that you can too.

First and foremost, you have to readjust your mental perspective. If your mind isn't right, your body won't be either. For example, I was in a spin class and my legs ached with that flu-like poison that permeates my limbs sometimes. In addition, my knees were making that arthritic cracking sound, which psychologically makes you cranky because you feel old and degenerating. After about five minutes, I didn't think I'd be able to continue because I felt annoyed and uncomfortable. There was a huge part of me that just wanted to sneak out and call it a day. My heart wasn't into it, and, apparently, neither were my legs. Then I scanned the room.

There is a woman that I've known for over twenty years who lost her entire leg to cancer. She is extremely fit and spins on a regular basis. I bet she would give everything she had to get her leg back. Who was I to piss and moan about my leg pain? At least I had two legs to bitch about. I almost succumbed to having a half-empty glass and that is not how I like to think. I finished the class and felt better after.

I had another incident at the gym that slapped me in the face the first time I witnessed it, and it continues to slap me on a regular basis. More importantly, it has given me perspective on my situation, preventing me from being a whiny bitch. One morning I was on the elliptical machine, and everything hurt. The pain brought tears to my eyes and I just wanted to quit. I was overtired and stressed out and my body was yelling at me. I knew that if I kept going, the endorphins would kick in at some point and I'd feel better. Still, the pain was real, and it was intense. Frankly, I felt defeated, discouraged, and pissed off. I kept my baseball cap low over my eyes to hide my tears as I scanned the room as a distraction. There was a man who lost both legs from the knees down in a boating accident walking on the treadmill near me with a big smile on his face. He works out regularly at the gym I go to. One day, I asked around to find out what happened to him. Apparently, he was boating with his family when one of his daughters fell off the boat, and when he jumped in to save her, the engine chopped off his legs. When I looked at him, I felt like an asshole. At least I had my legs to hurt. I kept going. Although our shit is real, there is always someone who has it a lot worse. That is how my mind works.

Recently I was taking a hot yoga class, and I had to modify my movements because my arms and neck were in so much pain. My hands were weak and numb, my elbow and shoulders were screaming at me, and my neck was stabbing and burning. That was when I noticed a new member of the class. It was a woman younger than me who only had one arm. Yep, time to stop being a whiny bitch, M.E., and find more gratitude. Do you see a pattern in how I think?

I briefly mentioned that my sister is gravely ill, but her cancer diagnosis is not new. Robin is only six years older than me and has had some shitty luck with her health. About twenty-five years ago, she was diagnosed with stage-three breast cancer at forty years old that spread to several of her lymph nodes. She had a mastectomy and had to undergo intense chemo and radiation therapy. She lost all her hair and was extremely sick during the treatment. It was obvious that the chemo was killing more than her cancer. It was unclear whether she would survive or not. This time was terrifying for all of us and, once again, it kept things in perspective. Cancer is a real disease that often takes our loved ones from us. Not that fibro isn't real, but I highly doubt that is what is going to kill me in the end. It was terrifying to watch her go through her ordeal, and our family is blessed she is still with us today. She is also the sister who has been given the grave diagnosis that her cancer has metastasized to her bones. We are trying to remain hopeful, and she is fighting it with everything she has, but it is so devastating. I am heartbroken.

No one should ever have to go through the nightmare she is living with right now.

But I also believe that if anyone can fight it, she can. She has four kids, eight grandchildren, and a fighting spirit, which is exactly what she needs. The doctors gave her a timeline on her mortality, which, in my opinion, is cruel and unforgiving. We have to have faith that she would defy the odds, and I know in my heart that if anyone can do it, she can.

I've always believed that your life will proceed in a direction based on how you look at things. If you focus on the notion that bad shit will always come your way, then it probably will. On the contrary, if you believe that tomorrow will be a good day, then it probably will be. I also think it is imperative to recognize how you react when bad things happen to you and also when bad things happen around you. Do you respond to stressors with negativity and anger, or do you try to keep your mind focused on a more rational and level-headed perspective? Essentially what I am asking you is whether or not your glass is half full or half empty. Mine, even with all of the shit that gets thrown my way daily, is half full. Negativity breeds negativity, and that is such an unfortunate way to spend what little time we have on earth. I'll never understand people who choose to be miserable. I truly believe that being miserable is a choice. I recognize that clinically depressed people have it harder than most, but there are also a ton of resources to help these individuals out as well. Even amidst illness and disease, you still have the ability to find some joy in your life. I may experience ongoing pain, nightmares, exhaustion, and even mental confusion, but it won't be the reason for my ultimate demise. It is a mantra I tell myself regularly. My sister could have died back then, and we are fortunate to still have her with us. Sadly, that shit spread, and it's not looking as hopeful, but who knows? I thank God that she was a survivor the first time around and I pray every day for a miracle. I can't compare my discomfort with what she went through and what she is going through now. Moreover, I can't even fathom how scared she must have been going through the surgery and all the subsequent treatments. It was a nightmare. And the nightmare is even worse now. So, I have fibromyalgia.

Big fucking deal. I'm the lucky one in my family.

Hands down, exercise has been my saving grace. As I mentioned earlier, exercise can be quite painful at times, but you need to be smart about it. I know that once the endorphins kick in, I can ride a bike, elliptical, treadmill, or rowing machine for an hour, and I'll feel amazing when the hour has passed. The first hurdle is to get your miserable ass out of bed and to the gym or to your basement where your fitness machines are collecting dust. Being sedentary is not your friend. I said it before, and I will say it again; motion is lotion. It's corny but true.

Let's take a quick moment to add a little science to this discussion. Did you know that when you perform cardiovascular exercises, there is a chemical called serotonin that is produced in the brain? Serotonin helps with mood and depression and makes you happier. If you're sitting around and not getting your heart rate up, chances are you're going to be as grumpy as Archie Bunker, a character in the 1970s TV show called *All in the Family* who complained a lot and rarely smiled. And if you're too young to remember that show, picture Oscar the Grouch from *Sesame Street*. He was pretty miserable, although he lived in a garbage can, so I guess I don't blame him for being a little grouchy.

One of your first hurdles is to make the conscious decision to start some kind of exercise program. You have to take that first step, which is always the hardest one. Remember, you have to walk before you run, so don't be too hard on yourself. If you get too ambitious, you could end up doing more harm than good. Be smart about whatever exercise program you decide to partake in. If you start slowly, you're less likely to become frustrated when things get really hard. The next difficulty is getting past those first ten minutes of an exercise routine when your body does not cooperate. Yes, my pain is real (especially when I start exercising), and I know yours may be too, but you can't let it win. Endorphins are more effective than any NSAID on the market and don't come with all the debilitating side effects. Let your body help you feel better. It's possible, I promise!

I have continued to keep some light weightlifting in my regime in spite of all my injuries. I admit that with all the tendonitis in my hands and arms and arthritis in my neck, back, and knees, it has been difficult. I can't do the same amount of weight I used to be able to do, and I can't weight lift for as long of a duration, but I still perform weight-resistance activities. I believe that staying strong helps me from getting even more injured, which almost sounds silly considering my current problems. Can you imagine if I didn't try to stay fit? I would be profoundly disabled and really fucking miserable.

Weight training also helps with controlling my weight. Science has proven that people who lift weights burn more calories at rest. Since extra pounds cause extra pressure on my joints, I'll lift those weights, even if they are really light. I want to burn as many calories as possible, especially while my body is adjusting to this annoying menopausal state.

A few years ago, I incorporated yoga into my workout regime. To say it has been a Godsend is an understatement. With my circulation issues, nothing is better than a hot yoga studio and fluid movement. You need to remember that being strong and flexible is essential to your well-being. Some days I kick ass in the yoga studio. On other days, I can barely do anything. The most important thing is that I SHOW UP. I don't stay in bed and whine about how shitty I feel. It doesn't make it better, so I continue to be proactive. And yes, active is an important part of that word. It isn't always easy, but it's as important as the air you are breathing.

As I've said over and over again, being inactive makes it worse. Movement is key. I have made a promise to myself to continually try to be proactive despite the poison and the pain. And once you figure out what cocktail works for you, the poison and pain just might be put on a back burner where it belongs.

I remember reading an article many years ago that talked about the best number of times a week you need to exercise to maintain your level of fitness, and what was needed to change it. It said that working out three times a week would help you maintain the weight and fitness level you are at right now. If you want to make a change, you need to go at least four or five times every week. In my situation, I strive for daily exercise, no matter how long or short of time I have. My commitment to a regular fitness schedule is no longer for maintaining my weight as much as it is to keep my body feeling better and my anxiety at bay. Since COVID, I no longer belong to a gym. Instead, I invested in workout equipment for my home. Making an investment in yourself is the best investment you can ever make. Exercise is vital to my well-being and should be vital to yours as well.

Weight control is a huge issue for fibro sufferers, and I totally understand how difficult it can be to maintain a healthy weight. Yes, we hurt. So, who the hell wants to work out when you are in pain? I get it, and it is something that I have dealt with also. However, I don't give in to it, and I don't want you to, either. The heavier I am, the more I hurt. It makes sense, doesn't it? It's a vicious cycle that can cause even more pain and depression. Extra weight puts extra pressure on your joints and tendons, and you can't afford to have unnecessary pressure on your body. It's exhausting to be unhappy in your own skin, so you need to figure out how to have control of your body as best as possible. Remember that excessive pounds will make it harder to do simple things, like walking up the stairs and watching your children or grandchildren. To make matters worse, many of the drugs prescribed for fibro patients cause you to gain weight. Now you're fat, and you're hurting. That's a shitty combo. And now that you're heavier, what's next? Probably depression. Maybe a little anxiety. Extreme exhaustion. Good times? Nope. You have to figure out a different strategy.

Now is the time to reiterate another monumental component in my fight against fibro that has helped me have control over how I feel—my diet. I realized over a decade ago that certain foods exacerbated my symptoms. As I said earlier in this book, beer, cooked tomato sauce, pasta, wheat, nightshade vegetables, processed foods, and fried foods make me miserable. Sadly, it took many years for me to realize there was a correlation, but I'm so glad I finally figured it out. It was uncanny how certain foods made me feel so much sicker. I realized that if I had spaghetti and meatballs for dinner, I would barely be able to walk up the stairs to go to bed at night. The pains and aches that traveled through my body were profound. One day I started paying attention to how I felt when I ate. It was a revelation like no other. I had figured out long before this those certain foods aggravated my system, but it seemed like a lot of work to avoid them. I wasn't ready to accept the fact that I couldn't eat whatever I wanted. Besides, I didn't want to make sacrifices when it came to food. I like food, and I like eating. I also don't like anyone or anything telling me I can't eat something, even if that somebody is ME! But when the realization hit me on the head, and I knew I had to finally pay attention.

Although I listed some of my trigger foods, that doesn't mean those foods are the same ones that will aggravate your system. Keeping a journal for a short period of time is a really good idea. You eat bread, and you feel bloated and gassy. Guess what? Gluten may not be your friend. I know your brain gets foggy, that's why it's important to write this stuff down. When you start paying attention to the cause and effect of what you eat and how you feel, you'll be amazed at the things you'll discover.

At one point I started a food blog because when I would post some of my recipes on social media, people were interested in the dishes I was making. It's called HungryHoo-Ha.blogspot.com, because everything I do seems to be hoo-ha related (again, the importance of a sense of humor must never be ignored). There are easy gourmet meals, including many gluten-free and vegetarian options. It's another avenue for me to share both my passion and what it takes for me to feel good.

Throughout my journey, I've studied a lot of alternative medicine. I've read countless books on nutrition and herbal remedies. Everything that I've read reinforces the notion that food is a big component in dealing with inflammation, pain, and illness. Even though I kept reading books and articles about the correlation between food and pain, I didn't follow through with changing my diet right away. I didn't want to believe that eggplant parmesan could wreak havoc on every part of my body, even though I knew it did. Don't get me wrong, I still eat it every once in a while. I just eat a smaller amount and can't be annoyed when I feel like crap after. I've tried many different diets throughout the years and have learned a lot. When the lightbulb finally went off in my head that I had to make changes in my diet, I contemplated getting a doctorate in wellness because I found the correlation between food and well-being so fascinating.

When I finally accepted the fact that my diet played a huge part in how I felt, I started making changes. I eliminated almost all beer from my diet, because it causes unusual abdominal distension and a throbbing ache in my limbs. If I want a beer, I usually have a Coronita, which is basically a half size bottle of Corona that my husband discovered for me years ago. That satisfies the craving but won't make me hurt. If I have more than one then I deal with the consequences, which are pretty uncomfortable and definitely not worth it.

If I want spaghetti sauce, I usually put it over escarole because the combo of sauce and pasta is deadly; unless it's gluten-free pasta like red lentil or black bean. Eggplant parmesan over pasta is hell because eggplant is considered a nightshade vegetable (which is not recommended for anyone with an inflammatory condition) and can do all sorts of nasty things to your system. Eggplant parmesan consists of cooked tomato sauce, pasta, *and* a nightshade veggie. It's a triple threat and a terrible combo for me. I love it, but it seriously does not love me. If I have the power to say no to foods that worsen the pain, why wouldn't I? As I said before, and I'll repeat until I'm blue in the face, you need to start a journal, because I'm confident you have foods that act like triggers also.

Once I realized that food could either help or hurt me, I started planning my meals even more conscientiously. Typically, I have a shake after I work out in the morning (with almond or cashew milk because dairy isn't my friend), a lunch that I prepare myself and take to work, and a balanced dinner. I try not to engorge myself at any meal because my body has difficulty digesting large amounts of food. I've also discovered that if I don't eat something every three to four hours, I get sluggish. Eating large amounts of animal protein also doesn't digest well. Five ounces is the maximum amount of steak or chicken that I can tolerate comfortably. You need to remember that everyone is different, so you have to figure out what works for you. I'm telling you what bothers me as an example for you to use when you assess your own diet.

Many fibro sufferers have problems sleeping, so we tend to get very tired. Caffeine is not the answer. For me, it revs up my heart rate, which makes me feel anxious. After my bout with panic attacks, I don't ever want to revisit that behavior again. It also dehydrates the body, and that can exasperate your misery—at least that is what it does to me. If you can handle the caffeine in green tea, go for it. It doesn't work for me because it makes me nauseous, but it could be your savior. Energy drinks are made with pure crap and are something you should avoid at all costs. I'll never understand why anyone would drink chemicals you can't even pronounce. I also stay away from soda and processed juices, because there is too much sugar in them. Ingesting chemicals and sugar with no nutritional value is very counterproductive to feeling better. Water, my friends, is vital to your well-being and can be life-changing if you currently have a lot of juices and sodas in your diet. I personally aim towards one hundred ounces. I recently heard you should drink half your body weight in ounces every day. That could work too. I know I need more because the hot flashes and working out make me dehydrated. One hundred ounces seems to be the number that works for me. Any less and I feel shaky, dizzy, and achier.

I'm sure you've heard that whole foods are best. Many people wonder what the expression "whole foods" even means. It basically means that you focus on eating fresh fruits and vegetables, not canned, boxed, or certain frozen ones. I freeze fresh fruit to use in my shakes.

For example, when bananas start getting brown, I remove the peel and put them in freezer bags. When strawberries get a little mold on them, I cut off the yucky parts and freeze them as well. I know a lot of people simply throw the fruit out as it gets old, but that is too wasteful. I also like to cut corn off the cob to freeze for my soups and stir-fry meals. Freezing your own food is a good idea, because then you know nothing has been added to it.

Eating better also means you eat real chicken and not chicken nuggets. Even if the nugget claims it is real white meat, it will still be covered with a coating of chemicals and sodium that are not good for you. To add insult to injury, that coating is fried, which is a means of cooking food that you should try to avoid. If you go to a local market, you'll find that eating with a whole-food mentality can be cheaper (and, hands down, it's a hell of a lot healthier). I try to buy my foods in bulk, as it's much more cost-effective. Anything I don't end up using, like organic chicken, I freeze in meal-sized portions for future use. It's also amazing to support your local farmers. They need the support more than the local supermarkets do.

Countless people freak out about their carbohydrate consumption because they are worried it'll make them fat. I do not believe that consuming carbs is the sole reason why people become overweight. Fast food, processed food, desserts, and the massive quantities of food people consume at one time are more likely the culprits that have led our society to be so obese.

For me, carbs make me feel crappy, so I have made the conscientious decision to limit the amount of them in my diet. If I'm really craving pasta or bread, I have a very small portion so it won't affect me as severely. I don't think feeling deprived is healthy, either. There is something about feeling deprived that can make you feel a little nutty and cause you to overindulge as a result of the deprivation. Furthermore, I don't think it is worth the bloat and ache that comes as the result of binging on any type of food. There is nothing glamorous about gluttony. It's funny, because I've never been a huge pasta or bread fan, but I married into an Italian family who believes you need bread with your pasta to soak up your sauce. Sadly, a lot of members of the family are overweight. Eating a lot of bread with pasta never made sense to me because it always made me feel too full. In fact, it makes me feel uncomfortably full, bloated, and pretty gross. I don't know why anyone would want to feel that way. You have to wonder if some people eat to live or live to eat. I suspect the latter.

I focus on lean proteins and fresh fruits and vegetables. When I eat something outside of those parameters, I suffer. It's as simple as that. "You are what you eat." Yeah, I believe that motto. It sounds simple enough, but I know it isn't. It's hard to say no to fried chicken and cornbread. I get it. I also know that I get sicker when I eat that kind of stuff, and the angst lasts a lot longer than the meal ever could. What I have to tell myself is that I may enjoy the fried chicken for ten minutes, but then I will suffer for hours and hours. You have to decide if it is worth it or not. On most occasions, I resist the temptation, because it isn't worth it.

Now is a good time in our society to try eating better. I think the massive obesity rate has changed the way we look at things. Countless companies are selling "clean-eating" plans. I don't think you necessarily need to invest in a plan unless you really need the guidance or the kick in the ass to stay motivated and on track. I'm thrilled people are talking about eating this way. It is a step in the right direction. It makes it so much easier to find the information that you need when more people are focusing on their health and wellness. If you need more information, ask Siri. It's amazing all the information that her sultry voice can give you. Or, in my case, my hunky male Australian Siri.

When I traveled to Italy for the first time a few years ago, I was blown away by how few overweight Italians I met. In fact, I'm not sure I met any. The people I encountered that were overweight tended to be Americans. I actually felt embarrassed by it. Are we really that careless about our health and well-being? Yes, I think we are.

Every restaurant we went to served real food. I never was served canned veggies or processed additives in anything I ate. I even ate pizza there and felt fine. They use real butter and extra virgin olive oil, not fake margarine, light oils, or any processed crap for that matter. Following a more European approach to eating is a smart idea. They never rushed us. We could spend two hours eating slowly and enjoying the fresh herbs, spices, and flavors that enhanced our meals. We also enjoyed one another, which was even more special.

Meal preparation and presentation are extremely important in Italy, and I was impressed by how much time and energy was put into their dishes. Since cooking has always been a hobby of mine, I appreciated all the thought and effort that the restaurants put into their meals. I enjoy planning and executing healthy and aesthetically pleasing meals and can appreciate what it takes to prepare a good meal. I also like to take my time to enjoy the food I've made. Getting a bacon cheeseburger, fries, and a Coke as I go through a fast-food restaurant drive-through is not my idea of a good food choice. They made food a priority and I, for one, appreciated it. None of the meals we ate were laden with excess calories, fat, or processed ingredients no one can pronounce. They eat well so they can live well. It was also so nice not to be rushed. More importantly, I enjoyed taking my time to savor a home-cooked meal with the people I love in one of the most beautiful countries in the world. There was no driving through Burger King and eating a Whopper on the way to the Vatican for this family.

Thank God my husband is supportive. For the most part, I don't want to eat carbs, so we have simply removed them from our diets. We usually have two veggies or a veggie and a salad with our protein with our meals. He has been such a champ. Not all men would be okay with that. When I don't eat carbs, I feel better. It's as simple as that. But if they are being served, I may get tempted to indulge. It's better to not have them around.

Let's take a minute to talk about what is fundamentally causing all this angst in our bodies and what techniques, aside from exercise and diet, that we can employ to feel better. It appears that fibro sufferers have an imbalance in our nervous system that makes us more sensitive to pain. In addition, our bodies and our brains are always living in that flight or fight mode. So, what is a good way to combat this panic in our bodies? We need to chill the fuck out. But even though we are exhausted, our bodies are too stressed out to relax and our brain continues to feel like it is swirling around in a fog of confusion? There are a lot of things that can help. For instance, I like to play words with friends daily. It keeps my mind focused on something besides my stressors and keeps my brain active. Maybe you prefer crossword puzzles or brain teasers. They all can help. Not only do you need to exercise your body, but you must also exercise your brain as well. On the other hand, you need to make time every day to relax your brain. Listen to calming music or meditation tapes is a great start. Breathing exercises like they do in yoga are also extremely beneficial for calming your nervous system down as well as helping you sleep, create more mindfulness, and lower your stress levels. I also like guided imagery. Close your eyes and go to a place that makes you happy. For me, I like to imagine the surf coming up on the sand in the ocean. I also like to imagine what I am like when I am pain free, fit, healthy, and most importantly, happy. And go outside. Staying inside for long periods of time can exasperate your depression and angst. There is nothing better than going for a walk in the woods or watching the sunrise. You do have options to feel better and now it's up to you to make it happen.

I would really like you to keep a journal so you can document your daily exercise, relaxation techniques, water consumption and food intake. It doesn't have to be forever, but at least until you realize what mental and physical exercises make you feel better and what foods aggravate your body. Is it dairy, gluten, or sugar? It may even be a combination of all three. The journal doesn't have to be fancy, thorough, or even neat. You could even use your phone. I want you to write down what you eat throughout the day, and then at the end of the day, think about how your body feels. Next, go about assigning each day a rating from one to ten. One referring to feeling shitty and ten referring to feeling fantastic. Or even better, draw a happy, sad, or ambivalent face. Whatever works for you is the way you should approach this task. It is essential that you figure out the connection between what goes in your mouth and how your body responds to it. I think you're going to be blown away when you realize what foods aggravate your system. And once you figure it out, it's up to you to find the willpower to stay away from them. I know that it can be hard, but I think living in constant pain is much harder.

You don't have to eat clean all of the time. That's unrealistic. But the cleaner you eat, the better you'll feel. Promise. Let me reiterate what that means. Stop buying things in cans and boxes. Ninety percent of your shopping list should be from the produce section and some from the butcher unless you're a vegetarian.

When my husband and I eat meat, we restrict our quantities. You don't need eight or ten ounces of steak. It's too much to digest. You'd be surprised how much better you'd feel if you only consumed four to six ounces of meat at a meal. I personally limit my protein consumption to four to five ounces. Even six ounces seems to be too much. When I see massive-sized steaks offered on menus at restaurants like the twenty-eight-ounce cowboy steaks, it makes me sick to my stomach. Our bodies were absolutely not made to consume that much meat. I don't know why anyone would think eating a small cow would be good for you.

Another biggie is to limit your dairy; it's hard to digest and tends to contain a lot of unnecessary and unhealthy fat. Recently, my doctor told me that my cholesterol was slightly elevated. He told me to stop eating so much ice cream. Ironically, I haven't eaten ice cream in years. The combination of sugar and dairy makes me bloated and usually gives me diarrhea. Am I lactose intolerant? I don't know. I'm not going to get tested. I just know that ice cream is not my friend. Listen to your body. It's telling you things and I'm pretty sure that you aren't being a good listener. I also prefer almond or cashew milk. Cow's milk gives me a stomachache, so it doesn't make sense to drink it. I didn't need a test to tell me what I instinctively know; if you get sick from eating something, then don't eat it.

I don't buy anything with the word diet in it. If I want butter, I use the real stuff—just not a lot of it. Those substitute products creep me out. Most of the time, I cook with olive oil anyways. If you read the ingredients in diet products, you wouldn't eat them either. Try to avoid eating things you cannot pronounce. It's a pretty simple rule. I'm convinced all the hormones and preservatives are making us sick. Cancer is everywhere, and girls are getting their periods at age nine. Don't tell me there isn't a correlation between all the diseases plaguing our society and our crappy diets. I blame the environment, too, but that's a whole other issue I don't want to get into.

Mark and I cook with a lot of fresh herbs that we grow in our garden and also ones that we buy from the store. They have incredible healing benefits and make food taste better. There are so many things that I make homemade because they're healthier and taste so much better.

Like salad dressing, for instance. I love homemade salad dressing. I make several different kinds. Most people who have my salad become addicted to it because the dressing is that good. That thrills me. Grocery store dressings have way too many ingredients in them that I have no idea what they are, except that they must be various forms of artificial chemicals to make the dressing last longer on the shelves. Is that what you want? Something that has enough preservatives in it to last a few years? I didn't think so. Disodium guanylate, disodium inosinate, and monosodium glutamate are just three examples of common ingredients found in many foods, including salad dressings. They sound super yummy, don't they? I would never ingest any of them unless they were completely natural, because those words frighten me. I have gotten to the point in my life where eating processed and unnatural ingredients grosses me out. Plus, they have a lot of unnecessary fat, sodium, and calories, which we don't need. Believe me, once you've made your own Caesar or Italian dressing, you'll be hooked.

Sugar is another ingredient you need to consume in extreme moderation. If you monitor how you feel when you eat a Snickers bar, I think you'll understand and agree with me that it should never be your snack of choice. You get a quick high and an even quicker low, which for someone like us can be quite debilitating. If you're a candy freak, consume the Halloween snack sizes and not a whole bar. And I mean only have one snack-size Snickers bar. Eating five small ones is equivalent to at least one large bar and completely defeats the purpose, although I know many people who reason that eating the small one's aren't quite as bad for you. I know it seems less if you eat a couple of small bars, but that's your mind playing tricks on you, and it isn't worth it in the end. It's like the client who brought me donut holes on a Saturday morning as a treat years ago. She told me there were no calories in them because they were the holes in the donuts. It was a clever thought, and her theory made me laugh. There was a part of me that thought she believed it. Donuts are not something I eat. If it looks good, I'll take a bite and leave it at that. Eating the whole thing would make me feel lousy, and it isn't worth it.

Stress is another component that can wreak complete havoc on your system. It would be foolhardy for me to suggest that you can have complete control of the stressors in your life. You can't and neither can I. But you can try to learn strategies to deal with your stress in a healthier and less detrimental way. Going to the gym helps me a lot. When I was in high school, I used to play the piano. I recently started playing again. I forgot how cathartic it could be. I also like puzzles. They are a great stress reliever that I highly recommend. Puzzles have saved me through some really dark periods in my life. Some people do yoga or meditate. I can't tell you what will work for you, but I can strongly urge you to figure something out. Agonizing over all the stressors in your life is not healthy. There are two things I need to remind myself of when I'm feeling anxious about a situation. First, will the issue be relevant one month, or even one year from now? In most cases, it won't. Secondly, you cannot control what other people do, say, or think, so stop obsessing over things you have absolutely no control over. That second statement has been a Godsend for controlling my anxiety, personally and professionally.

I have discovered that writing has been one of my most important saving graces. To date, I've written a very funny nonfiction collection about my career called *The Happy Hoo-Ha Trilogy*. I recently finished writing the fifth book in a fictional erotic romance series called *A Promise of Passion*. I've started a sexy fictional book loosely entitled *Sexy in Scrubs*, which is a funny and naughty book about a young woman in medical school. I keep a blog called *Hose Down Your Hoo-Ha*, which I've been writing since 2010 about my crazy career as a Brazilian wax technician. I've made a concerted effort to blog every day. In fact, I've missed very few days over the past decade. Writing is a great way to focus on something besides my ailments. It also gives my body a chance to rest since I am such a high-strung person who is always on the go. It's also a great distraction from all the serious things in our lives. No matter what I am writing, it takes me away. Letting your mind be creative and go to someplace fun can be as therapeutic as a walk on the beach or a two-hour massage.

I guess one of the most important lessons I can teach you is to listen to your body, which I have repeated time and time again in this book. Sometimes, I don't pay close enough attention to what I eat or drink because it can be a pain in the ass to focus on everything I ingest. But when I realize I feel crappier than usual, I'll reflect on what I put in my mouth that day or the night before and also what kind of stressors I had to deal with. Usually, there is a correlation, and it's important to figure out what pissed your system off. If I have eaten really well and there is still a flare-up, then it is usually stress or injury related. Be aware of what is happening in your life and in your body. You are the captain of your personal vessel, and it is time to take charge of that miraculous vessel so that you can drive through calmer waters.

What I'm suggesting requires some thought and planning, but it isn't as daunting as you might think. Thinking and strategizing about exercise, diet, and stress is necessary if you want to find some relief, but it does take some time. Since your brain can hold an infinite amount of information, I'm going to suggest the absolute most important component that you need to concentrate on in order to be happy—your mind. It is *imperative* that you adopt the most positive mindset possible, or you will never be able to move forward. I know that it can be nearly impossible some days, but you have to persevere. You've read about all the crap I've had to deal with, and I have never and will never give up my quest to live as pain-free and as happy as possible. It's overwhelming to live in chronic pain, and there are times that I have a really intense cry, but that is okay too. You are human, and having health issues can be daunting and downright exhausting, but you have to find the light. I'm assuming your issues are overwhelming as well or you wouldn't be interested in a book like this. I know that the pain can be crippling, and there are many of you that will be forced to stop working, but you can still find joy in your life. I know you can. You have to truly believe that you *deserve* to be happy and make a plan to do just that.

One of my suggestions is that you read an inspirational book. I found the book *The Secret* extremely liberating because it is important to fill your mind with positive stories. There are people who have lived through stage-four cancers and have walked after spinal injuries. Wouldn't you like to be that person who was truly able to overcome your physical limitations and be able to perform tasks that you never thought possible? Lamenting about your ailments isn't helping, so try to think about your innate power to help yourself. It may sound a little corny to some of you, but let me ask you this, what do you have to lose?

I believe that it is vital to do your homework about your disease or your specific ailments.

Knowledge is so powerful. Don't be complacent and simply accept your doctor's instructions. Remember the story about my knee issue in high school? One doctor told me to sit in a wheelchair for six months, and the next one told me to get my ass up and start weightlifting. There are two approaches—be complacent or be proactive. I guess the wheelchair incident changed my perspective more than I ever knew. I'm no longer complacent. I don't think you should dismiss your doctor's directive, however. Take all of their advice and formulate a plan that works for you. I respect my doctor, but I don't agree that taking Neurontin or Lyrica is the answer for me. You know your body better than anyone. It's time to take control.

Many people have to take medication because of a given ailment that requires it, like diabetes, epilepsy, or MS, and in those instances, I hope you all find a prescription that helps your symptoms and makes your situation better. What I would like you to consider is eliminating some of the medications that are causing all of those horrific side effects that you may not actually need. I know that certain medications can be absolutely necessary to your ability to function, but you may be surprised how much better you feel if you take less or even go drug-free. Most people are completely shocked that I don't take any prescription medications considering all the things wrong with me. They don't help. They just make me have other issues.

No thanks, I'll pass.

More than anything, I want you to be proactive about being happy. Grab this obscure disease by the balls and show it who's boss! You have so much more power over your well-being than you're giving yourself credit for. I'd like to suggest that you might have just forgotten that notion because your brain got foggy from the drugs you've been taking. That's okay. I'm here to give you permission to try to eliminate some of the fog and to find more joy in your life.

There is something else I really want you to do. I want you to laugh more. I have integrated a lot of laughter into my profession, and it has made all the difference in the world. Maybe it isn't possible for you to laugh a lot at your job, but that doesn't mean you can't find new ways to laugh some more in your personal life. Watch funny movies. Go to a comedy club. Read funny books. They say, "An apple a day keeps the doctor away." I think laughter is as important as that proverbial apple. And if you can laugh so hard that snot runs out your nose, even better. There is nothing better than some nasty boogers to highlight your day and bring sunshine to your soul.

You have to believe that you have some control of your destiny. Let that be another one of your mantras that you tell yourself so many times, it actually becomes a reality. You also need to remember that this is rarely a fatal condition. That simple (but ginormous) fact makes all the difference in the world to me. If I get cancer one day, I may not be able to say the same thing. But for now, I can. I have to look at the positive side of all of this. I may not be able to smile away my fibro, but smiling most definitely makes it more bearable. Believe me, the more joy you can find in your life, the easier it'll be to deal with your symptoms.

You only have one life and one body. It is up to you and you alone to treat it well. Believe in yourself and your power to make a change. I'm going to say it again and again and again: don't be complacent with the doctor's diagnosis unless you are sure that their diagnosis, suggestions, and treatment plan are exactly how you think this game should be played. Our body is incredible at healing itself if you let it. I may not be able to control the disease, but I can control the symptoms with some concentrated effort and a positive attitude.

Make a specific plan and set goals for yourself. Whether you incorporate some form of exercise (which I pray you do), change your diet (which I'm also praying you do), or reintroduce hobbies that make you happy, you have to make yourself a priority. If you are able to make yourself a priority, you will be happier. I truly believe this. When you are happier, the people around you will be happier as well. Smiling is infectious, as is laughter and joy. Being grumpy can also be infectious, but it isn't as fun, and I don't recommend it—ever. Being depressed isn't making your life complete, so let's try another approach.

Choose a better life for yourself, and you and your loved ones will all reap the benefits. I know you want more out of life. So do I. That is why I've made a conscious effort to make the most out of every day and to think positively no matter what. Don't succumb to the textbook definition of the label that has been put on you. I don't fit the criteria of a typical fibro patient because I refuse to let it define me. Being overweight, lethargic, and depressed is not an option. All three of those conditions will make me miserable, and frankly, I don't want misery to be in my company. Stop making it an option for you. I will fight it until the day I die and so should you. I feel like I've wasted a lot of time seeing doctors and lamenting over this label they have attached to my name. It's exhausting trying to deal with the myriads of problems that keep arising, but since that is what I keep experiencing, then I've been forced to be as proactive as possible with my health.

Every morning I try to focus on what I need to do to get my ass out of bed, make myself feel better, and have a great day. Through a lot of reading, planning, and self-awareness, I have figured out how to have a fulfilling life, and I believe in my heart of hearts that so can you. How you approach every day is totally up to you, my friend. You can choose to be miserable or choose to be happy. It really is as simple as that.

So, when you wake up tomorrow morning, and the pain and exhaustion are consuming every molecule of your body, I want you to do me a favor. Get out of bed and say, "Fuck you, Fibro!"

Thanks for your time!

Love and sunshine,
M.E.

www.ingramcontent.com/pod-product-compliance
Lightning Source LLC
Chambersburg PA
CBHW070832160726
48004CB00001B/341